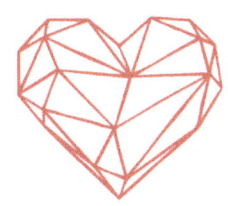

RECLAIMING POSTPARTUM WELLNESS

Maranda Bower

Reclaiming Postpartum Wellness

A HOLISTIC GUIDE TO RETURNING TO THE
ROOTS OF HEALTH IN MOTHERHOOD

Maranda Bower

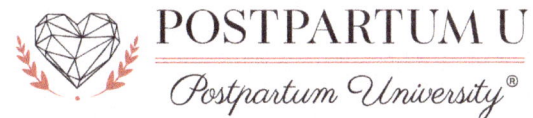

CONTENT PRESENTED IN THIS BOOK OR OTHERWISE IS NOT A SUBSTITUTE FOR PROFESSIONAL MEDICAL ADVICE, DIAGNOSIS, OR TREATMENT OR A PROFESSIONAL, THERAPEUTIC RELATIONSHIP. CONTENT PRESENTED IS INTENDED TO PROVIDE GENERAL HEALTH INFORMATION FOR EDUCATIONAL PURPOSES ONLY. IT SHOULD NOT BE USED AS A SUBSTITUTE FOR MEDICAL OR PSYCHIATRIC ADVICE, CANNOT DIAGNOSE OR TREAT ANY MEDICAL OR PSYCHIATRIC CONDITION, AND DOES NOT REPLACE CARE FROM YOUR PHYSICIAN. You should not rely on content presented in this book or any program offered or associated with Postpartum University® for diagnosis or treatment of any health condition. We are not healthcare professionals or providers. Always consult a healthcare professional if you suspect you require medical or psychiatric treatment. If you believe or suspect you are experiencing an emergency, call 911 immediately (or your local emergency hotline).

ALL RIGHTS RESERVED. This book contains materials protected under International and Federal Copyright Laws and Treaties. All information in this publication is strictly for informational purposes only and should not be taken as medical advice. By reading and using this document, you agree to abide by the copyright policy and only use this publication for personal informational use and not as a substitute for medical or other professional advice. This book and its contents are not to be shared with anyone. Distribution of this book is under exclusive licensing rights of the distributor. To share this information, refer to www.PostpartumU.com with information on where to purchase.

If you have any questions about the rights of sharing our content, do not hesitate to contact us. We really appreciate your understanding.

RECLAIMING POSTPARTUM WELLNESS, Copyright 2022, by Maranda Bower.
All rights reserved. Printed in the United States of America.

www.PostpartumU.com

The Library of Congress has cataloged the paperback edition as follows:

Title: Reclaiming Postpartum Wellness
Names: Maranda Bower, author
Description: Alaska, 2023 | Includes bibliographical references and index.
Identifiers: LCCN: | ISBN: 979-8-9878476-8-8 (paperback)

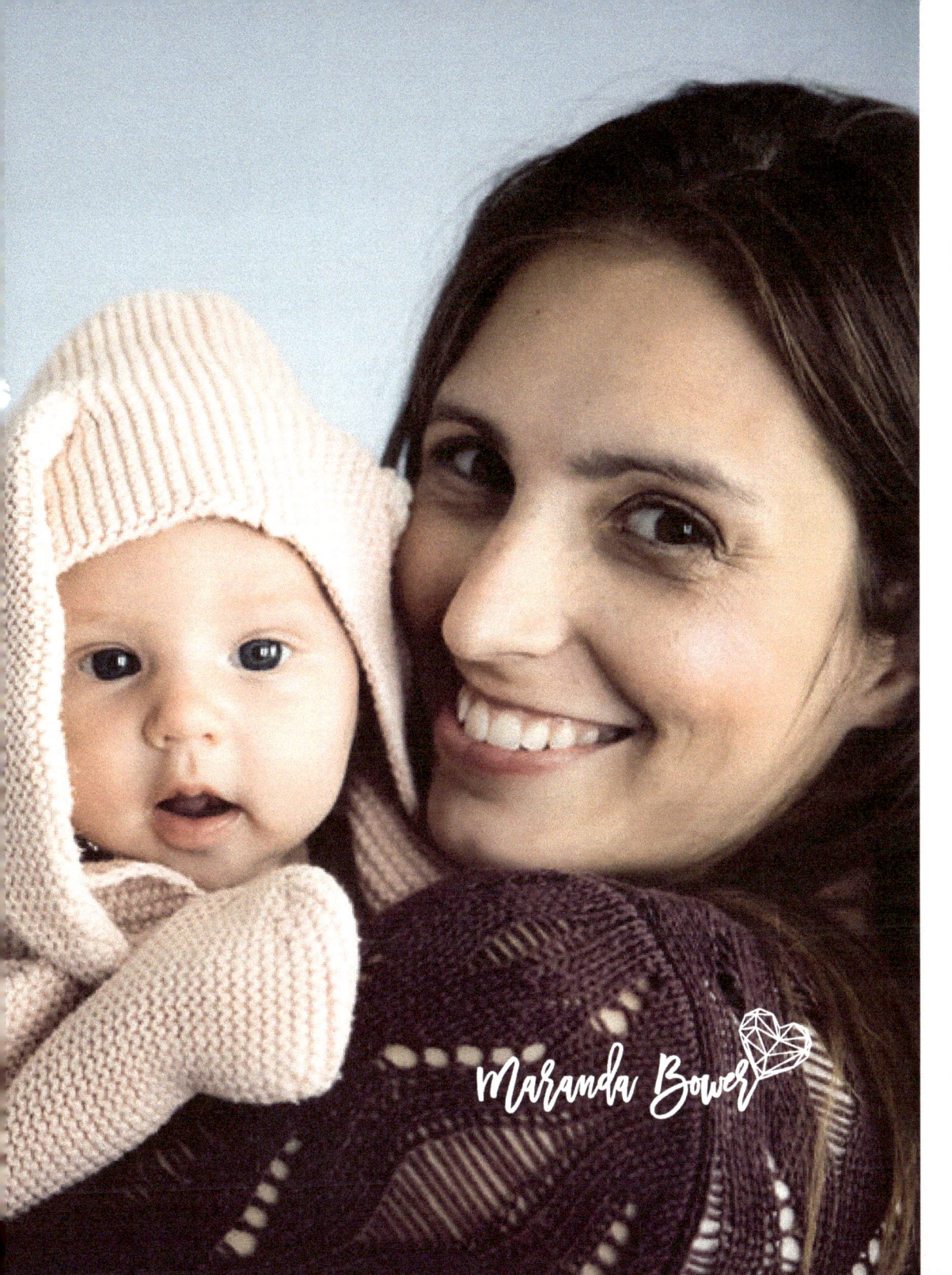

Reclaiming Postpartum Wellness

A holistic guide to returning to the roots of health in motherhood

Maranda Bower

Dedicated to my 4 beautiful children.

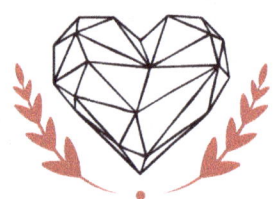

Content

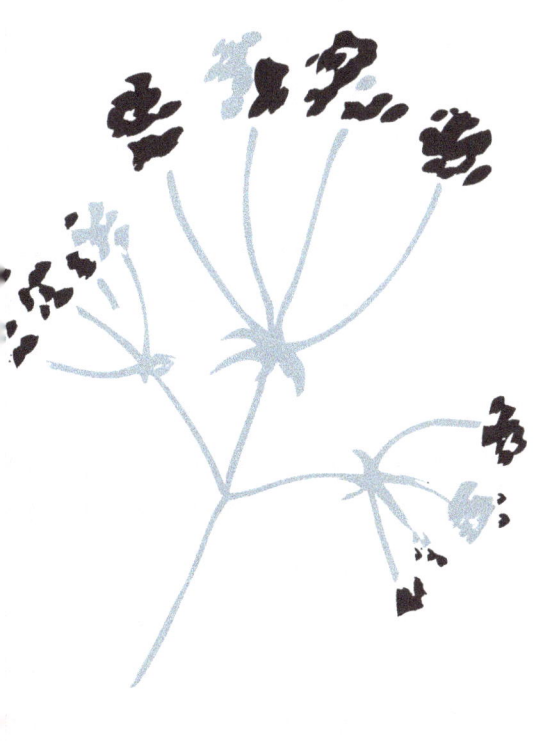

Dear Mama — 1

Introduction — 3

Chapter 1: Support — 18

Chapter 2: Nutrition — 37

Chapter 3: Sleep — 59

Chapter 4: Nervous System — 72

Chapter 5: Rhythms — 102

Chapter 6: Movement (Bonus) — 109

Glossary of Terms — 123

Acknowledgments — 129

Additional Resources — 130

References — 131

Dear Mama,

Motherhood is filled with both beauty and peril. It brings you love beyond measure and challenges that you could never anticipate. The act of mothering has been created for our greatest growth; to stretch us to the heavens and into the hands of all that is. But that stretch in today's modern world often feels more like a painful tug-and-pull war.

Whatever you are feeling, you are not alone. My own experiences in motherhood were marked with depression, anxiety, rage, autoimmune disease, and even postpartum bipolar disorder. Through 4 children, I have truly understood what it means to feel as if my body was broken, that I was too difficult a case to heal, and that life was simply spiraling to an uncontrollable end.

There are depths to my stories (as there are within yours) that could fill another book altogether. But rather than these stories becoming my demise, they've instead pushed me to a greater understanding of what is not only possible in this world, but also what is greatly needed in order for our families to live better.

Through my own journey of healing in motherhood, I learned more about myself and my abilities as a mother, woman, and human being. I studied everything related to motherhood that I could possibly study. I went back to school, signed up for numerous certification programs, attended conferences when I could, and witnessed and supported births. I soaked up every bit of knowledge and energy I could, forcing myself to practice another way of life (as I'm showing you within these pages) until I could breathe again. Until I could sense that I was, indeed, going to do more than just survive.

In those years, I wrote books, spoke at Universities and conferences around the world, held classes, founded Postpartum University®, and now run the most distinguished postpartum nutrition program (along with many other programs) on the globe, focusing on bringing holistic, traditional medicine together with evidence-based science to support whole-body healing at its very core. I did it all so that mothers can heal, thrive, and love life with kids.

Today, I have known and supported thousands of women through the common symptoms of:

- Depression/ anxiety
- Major hair loss
- Exhaustion/ fatigue
- Recurring headaches
- Aching joints or muscle pains
- Irrational and intrusive thoughts
- Period pain and mood swings
- And so much more…

If you take one thing away from this book, let it be that you are never alone. You are worthy of good health, and there is nothing more magnificent and divine than motherhood. You can feel good again with the right tools. There is a great reason for you finding this book.

Welcome. I am so glad you are here.

Introduction

You'll learn:

- Root Cause Care
- Steps to Postpartum Wellness
- Postpartum Facts
- Breaking Cycles
- Postpartum Changes

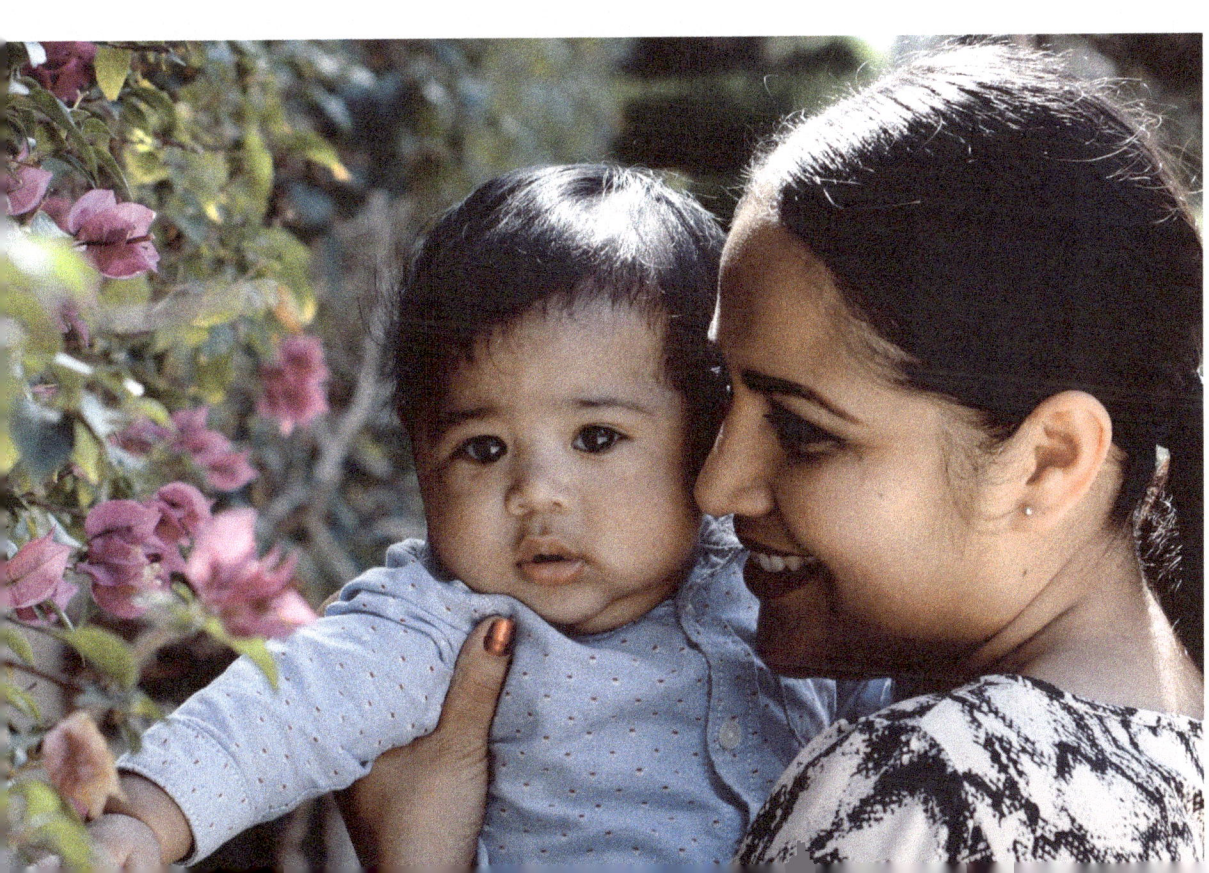

The Beginning

Roots of Postpartum Wellness

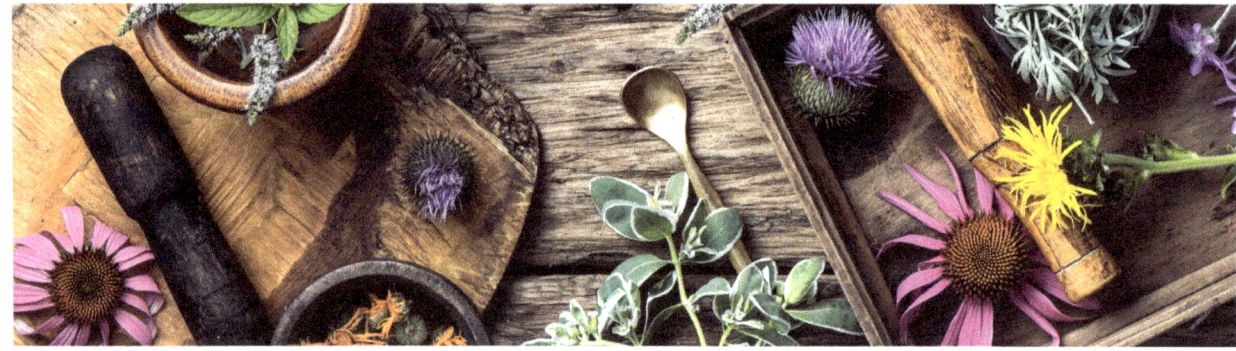

One of the biggest medical myths is that the body functions in separate parts rather than as a whole. In postpartum, the physiological and psychological shifts temporarily redefine digestion, absorption, thinking, and immune function. This impacts every aspect of the body. It all works together.

Root Cause Care recognizes that an imbalance that is usually generated in postpartum creates long-lasting symptoms that have been labeled as "normal." Depression, anxiety, bloating, fatigue, major hair loss, hormone imbalance, depletion, autoimmune issues, organ dysfunction, and so much more are all too common but far from normal.

In this book, you'll learn an evidence-based framework (Your Steps to Postpartum Wellness) to supporting your body at its foundational roots, helping prevent and eliminate these symptoms while creating balance and health.

Your Steps to Postpartum Wellness

Understanding how your body functions and how to support it is important, but having actionable tools is critical and life-changing. When you follow these steps in the order that they are presented here and apply the information, you'll be on your way to whole-body healing.

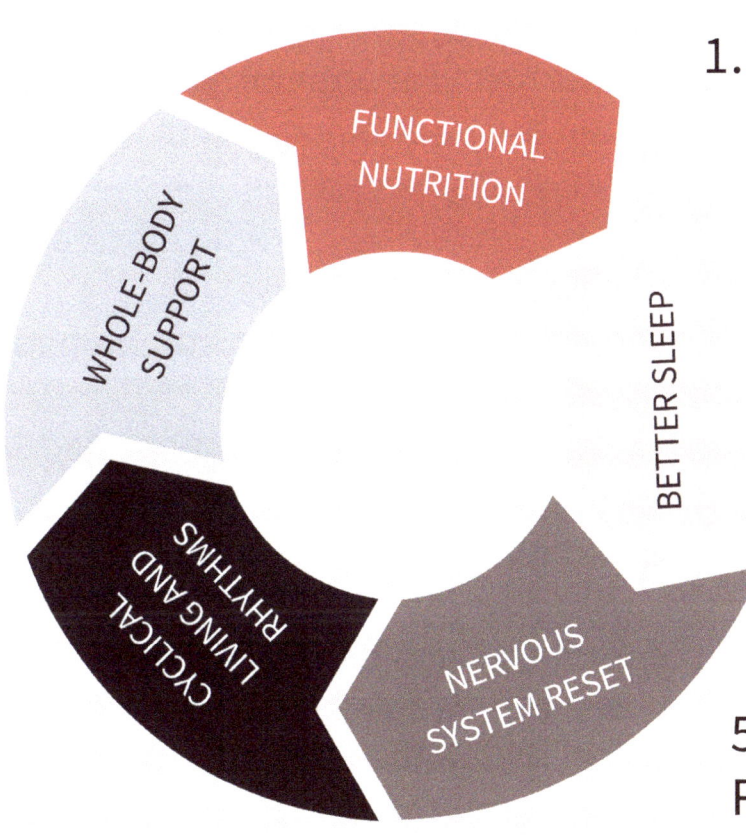

1. Whole- Body Support

2. Functional Nutrition

3. Better Sleep

4. Nervous System Reset

5. Cyclical Living and Rhythms

Let's talk facts.

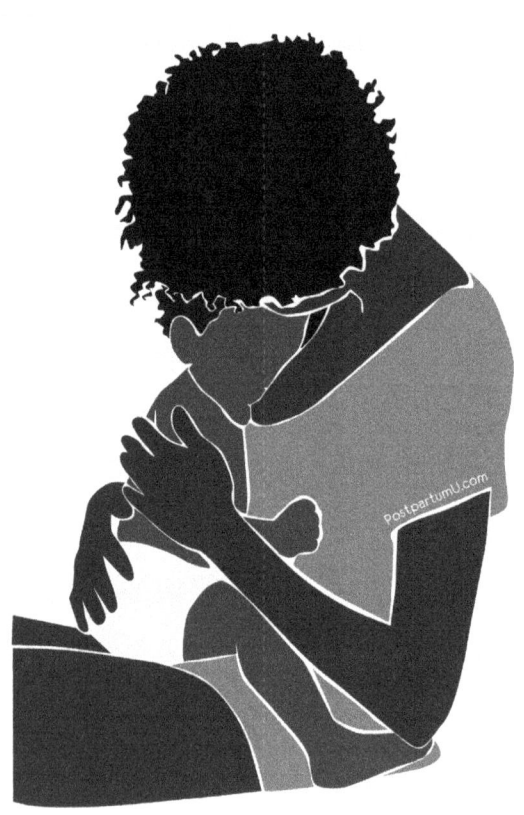

- 7 out of every 10 women are prescribed medications in pregnancy.
- More than 30% of women in postpartum will be diagnosed with a mental health disorder and rates are rising.
- Women are at a 28% increased risk of developing a postpartum autoimmune disease in the first year after birth.
- 1 in 7 women will be diagnosed with a thyroid disorder.
- Babies are suffering from increased childhood illnesses and disease.
- Dysfunction and imbalances in motherhood are being labeled "normal."
- Women feel they are not fully supported in whole-body healing and that something major is missing from their overall care.

These statistics are unable to account for those who don't feel safe sharing their experience, those who aren't aware of a problem until the fog of it begins to clear, or for those who don't feel it until they begin to wean from breastfeeding or when the menstrual cycle returns a year or more after birth.

If we look at these numbers and facts, what we see is an epidemic. We are witnessing a universal crisis.

And we need to ask the question: WHY IS THIS HAPPENING? How is our society failing mothers? What is it that we don't know? And more importantly, how can we better support healing?

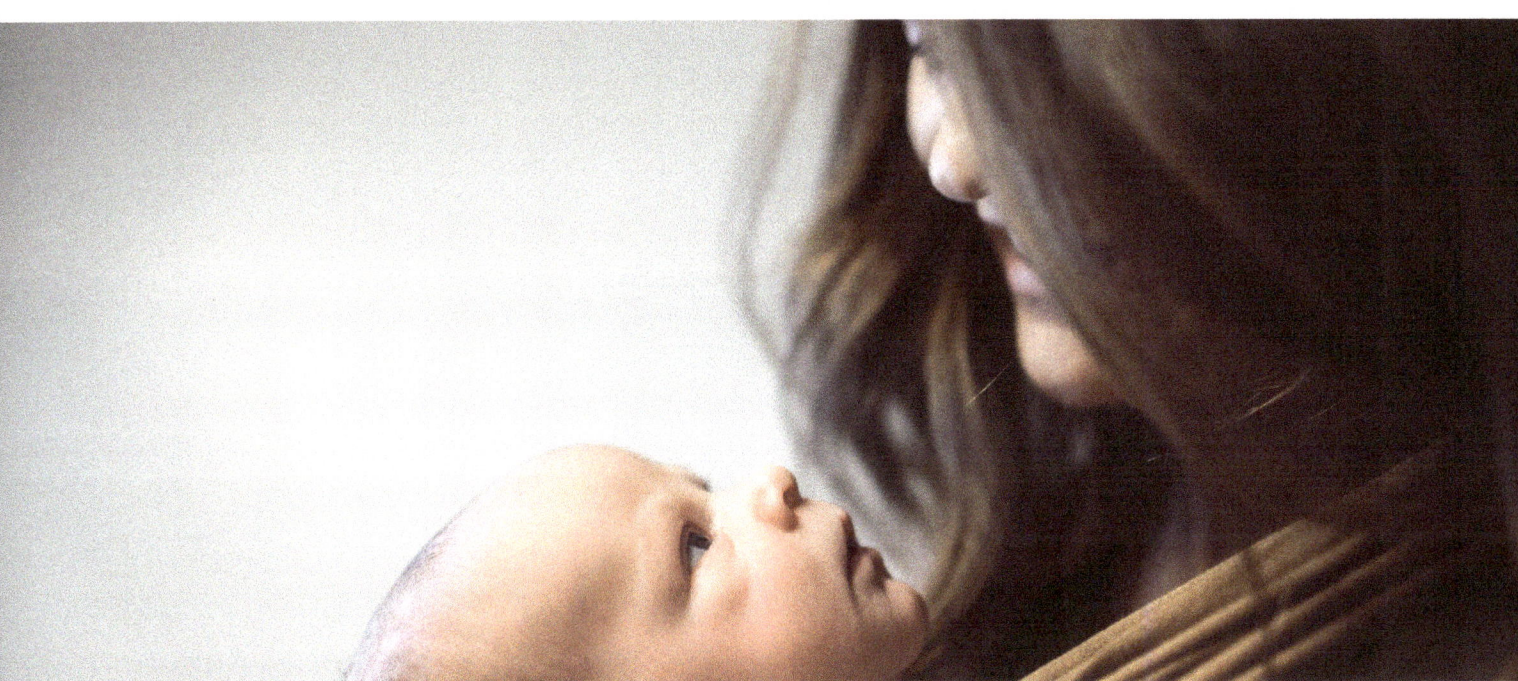

You are not broken because you have a baby, and you do not need to settle for mediocre motherhood. It's time to reclaim your postpartum wellness.

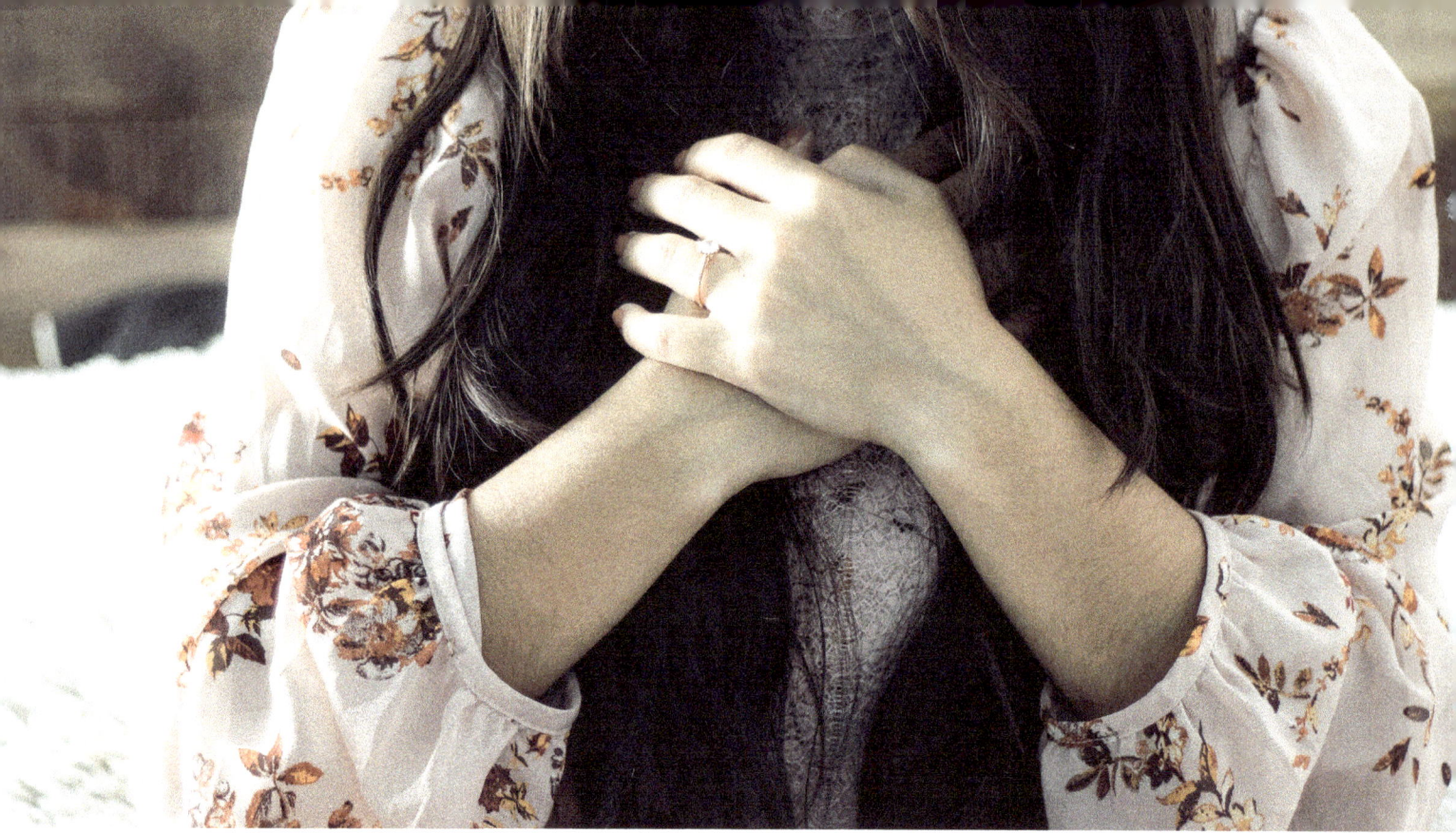

When you aren't feeling well physically, mentally, and emotionally...

...it will greatly compromise your well-being, your parenting, and your life.

This has lasting repercussions on you as well as your family and community.

The health of a community begins with its mothers.

So, let's get you better starting now.

Getting healthy isn't a quick fix. It's a lifestyle shift.

In today's modern world, we've placed value in fast results and constant forward motion that involves everything but rest, reflection, and supportive health practices.

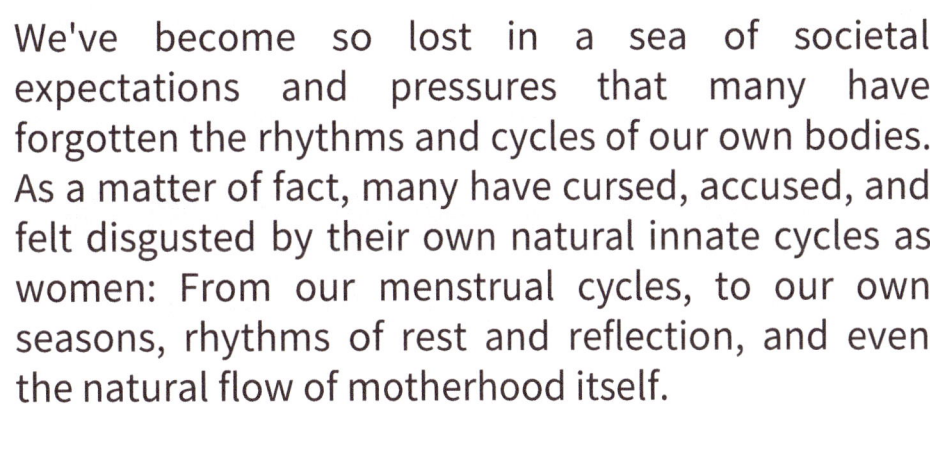

Only when life feels unbearable do we stop for a single second to incorporate a quick fix, just to return afterward to the busyness and chaos of life that created the need for critical care and support in the first place.

This lifestyle is the source of much dysfunction, disease, and dysregulation.

We've become so lost in a sea of societal expectations and pressures that many have forgotten the rhythms and cycles of our own bodies. As a matter of fact, many have cursed, accused, and felt disgusted by their own natural innate cycles as women: From our menstrual cycles, to our own seasons, rhythms of rest and reflection, and even the natural flow of motherhood itself.

Health practices are interwoven into our lives. It is only when we return to the roots of our body and these innate rhythms that we will be able to restore an instinctual, intuitive, balanced state of health, well-being, and ease.

3 Pillars of Knowledge

Throughout this book, I will be walking you through holistic, traditional medicine and spiritual guidance and techniques that are supported by evidence-based science, tradition, and women's stories from around the world.

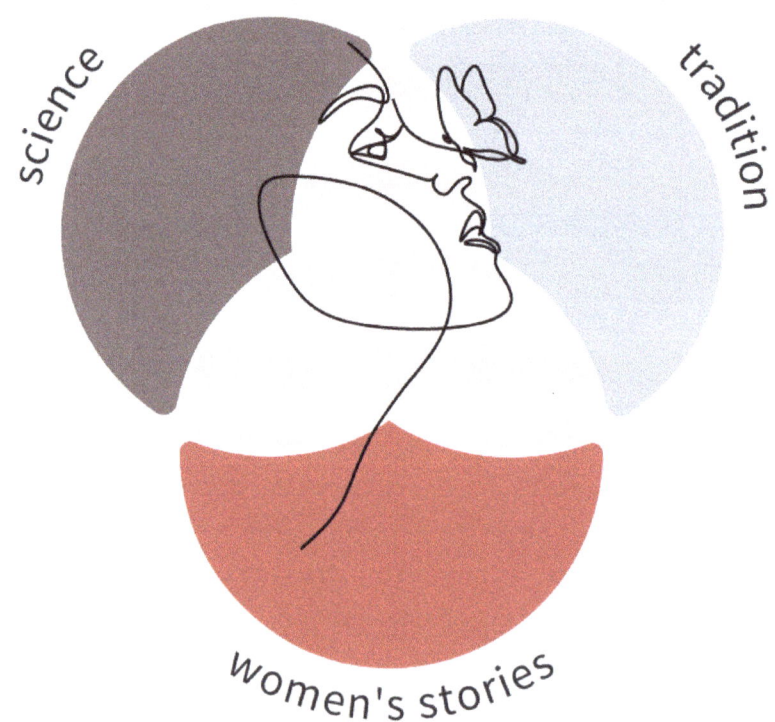

These 3 pillars of knowledge are necessary to support a whole-body approach to care and healing. Without one, our information will be greatly limited. Together this creates a recipe for strength, vitality, and conscious care in motherhood.

When you understand the inner workings of your body, you are able to apply more specific healing techniques that get to the root of your needs.

Breaking the Cycle and Returning to Your Roots

Reclaiming your own personal rhythms requires five major changes within your life: support, nutrition, sleep, nervous systems tools, and following your natural rhythms, all of which are covered in detail in this book. In postpartum, these Roots to Healing are the foundations of living. These are what need to be a part of your everyday life.

> This book exists to break down barriers, bring you back into your body, and support you in creating more meaning, ritual, and healing throughout your life.

In order to get to that place of joy and well-being, the walls and blockades to your health have to be addressed in full. Many mothers I work with wait until the very last minute, when the pain is tremendous, before reaching for support or advocating for their needs. As our body sends us warning signs such as depression, anxiety, hair loss, mood swings, fatigue, gut problems, and more, they are generally ignored, covered up with medications or temporary health care, or downplayed as normal parts of motherhood. Once these symptoms are addressed fully using the Roots to Healing, then the layers of dysfunction, dis-ease, and dysregulation can begin to fall away. From there, the unraveling of wellness will blossom.

Health and well-being are the normal states within your body. Anything outside of wellness are signals for you to re-calibrate, realign, and reassess your daily life. It is your innate right to feel good in your body.

Long ago, postpartum practices were designed to support women in finding and fine-tuning their health as a mother. The knowledge and power of these traditional postpartum wisdoms have been lost from our modern world. As a consequence, postpartum mothers are experiencing a significant amount of emotional, mental, and physical pain - and it's considered normal.

It's time to Reclaim Postpartum Wellness.

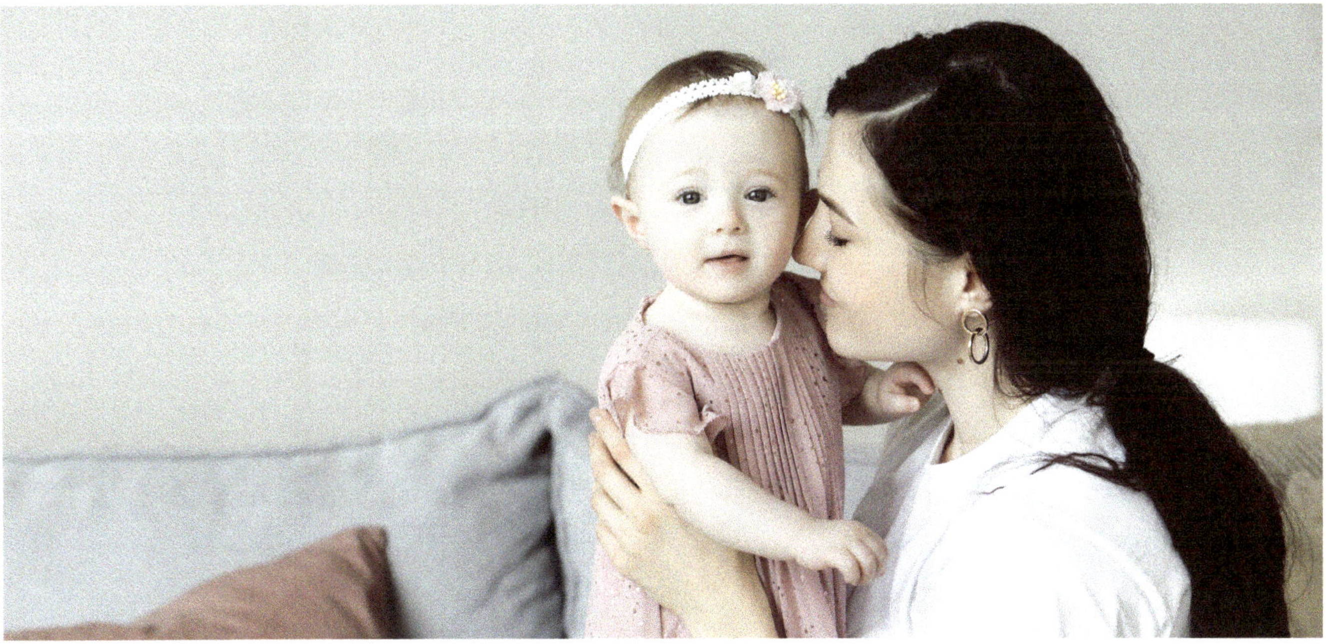

Back to the Roots

What You Need to Know

Every single practice presented in this book is rooted in both modern life and tradition, a blend between science and sacred. Without telling the story of the postpartum traditions around the world, we lose the connection from our ancestors and the mothers who've come before us. Without their stories and wisdom, we would have nothing more than meaningless jargon on paper. Science is only a mere fraction of the evidence needed to support the practices shared with you here, and it has a long way to go in order to catch up to the intelligence and validity of ancient traditions.

In order to change the way we experience postpartum in this modern world, we must connect with our ancestral mothers and go back to our roots.

Your body is physiologically and psychologically different for many months and years after birth.

This means that your nervous system, your gut function, and your mental processing all operate differently than they did in pregnancy and before.

How your body senses danger, digests foods, expresses love, and its needs for healing have changed. Many of us recognize that our body has transformed on a physical level. But the shifts that occur within are less understood or even spoken about.

This book exists to bring light to these physiological and psychological transformations that affect every postpartum woman and to support deep healing in the process. When you understand the inner workings of your body, you are able to apply more specific healing techniques that get to the root of your needs. This translates to faster and more profound healing and well-being.

Created from a culmination of science, collaboration, cultural study, and countless interviews and the experiences of hundreds of women over the course of a decade of research, this is explicitly for you.

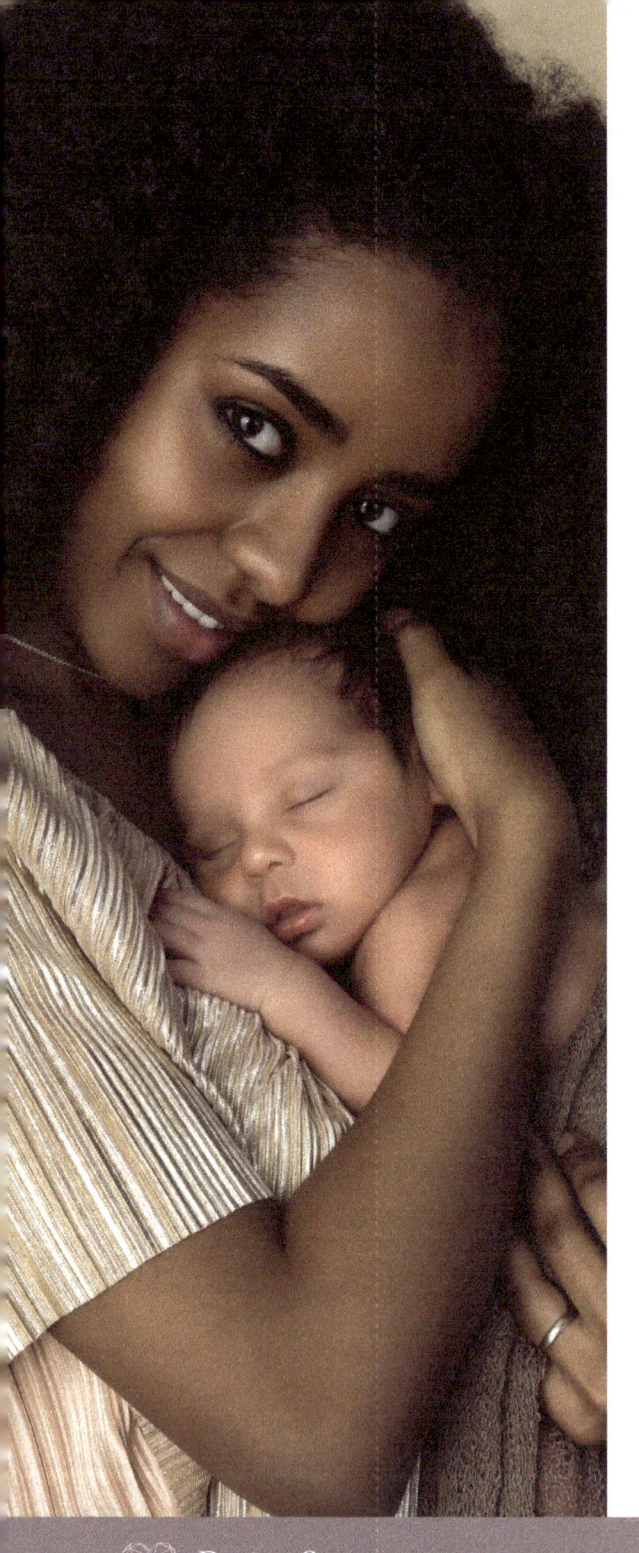

Postpartum is not the first 6 weeks after baby. It's the first 6 years.

How you experience this monumental life change will shape your life forever. Your healing (or lack thereof) will impact your entire life, including your menopause.

Postpartum also shapes the way your baby and children experience life. When you aren't well, you connect with them differently. Their understanding of life, and how to cope with challenges, will be greatly determined by you.

Let's not forget partners. Divorce rates are highest in the first year after birth. Your child's initiation into parenthood is influenced by you.

The saying "if a mama isn't happy, no one is" exists because of its truth. **In other words, your wellness is incredibly important, not just for you but for your entire family.**

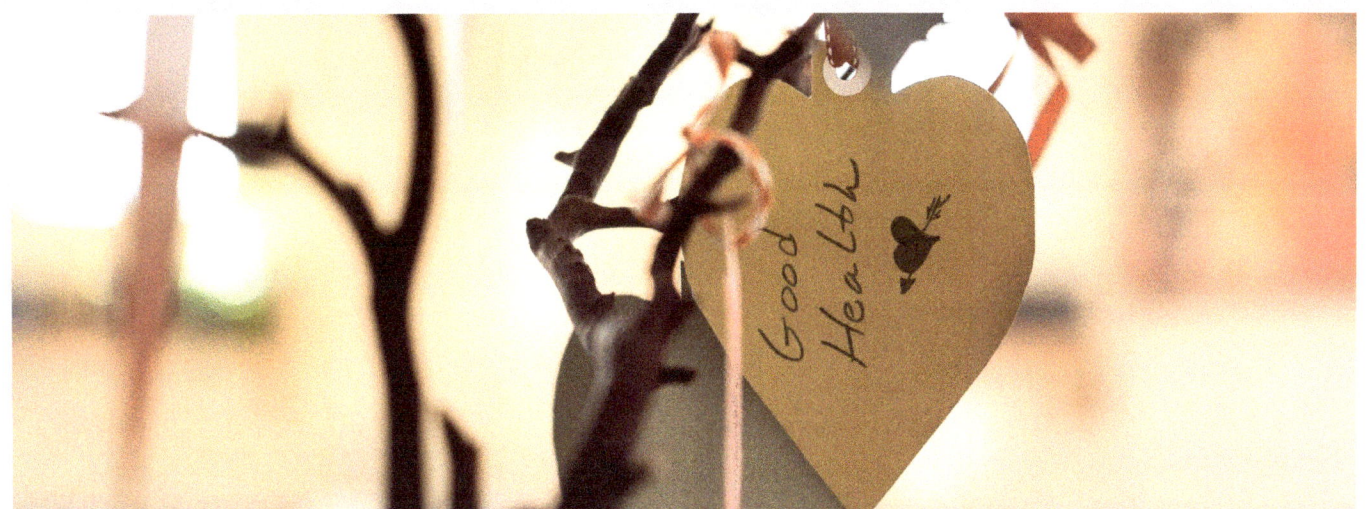

It's never too late to heal.

No matter where you are in your postpartum journey, or how many years post-birth you are, the healing techniques I'm sharing with you in this guide are applicable to you. They are also amazing healing methods you can use with your family, especially when one isn't feeling well.

Each section in this guide is incredibly interrelated. You cannot experience a deep transformation without all of these components, even though you can easily feel the benefits of each one without the other.

In order to maximize your healing, incorporate some or all of the practices mentioned in every section into your daily life. By doing so, you will create a strong foundation within you in which all things will reverberate.

1. Support

You'll learn:

- Real Support
- The Path of Healing
- Steps to Getting Support
- Taking Assessment

Chapter One

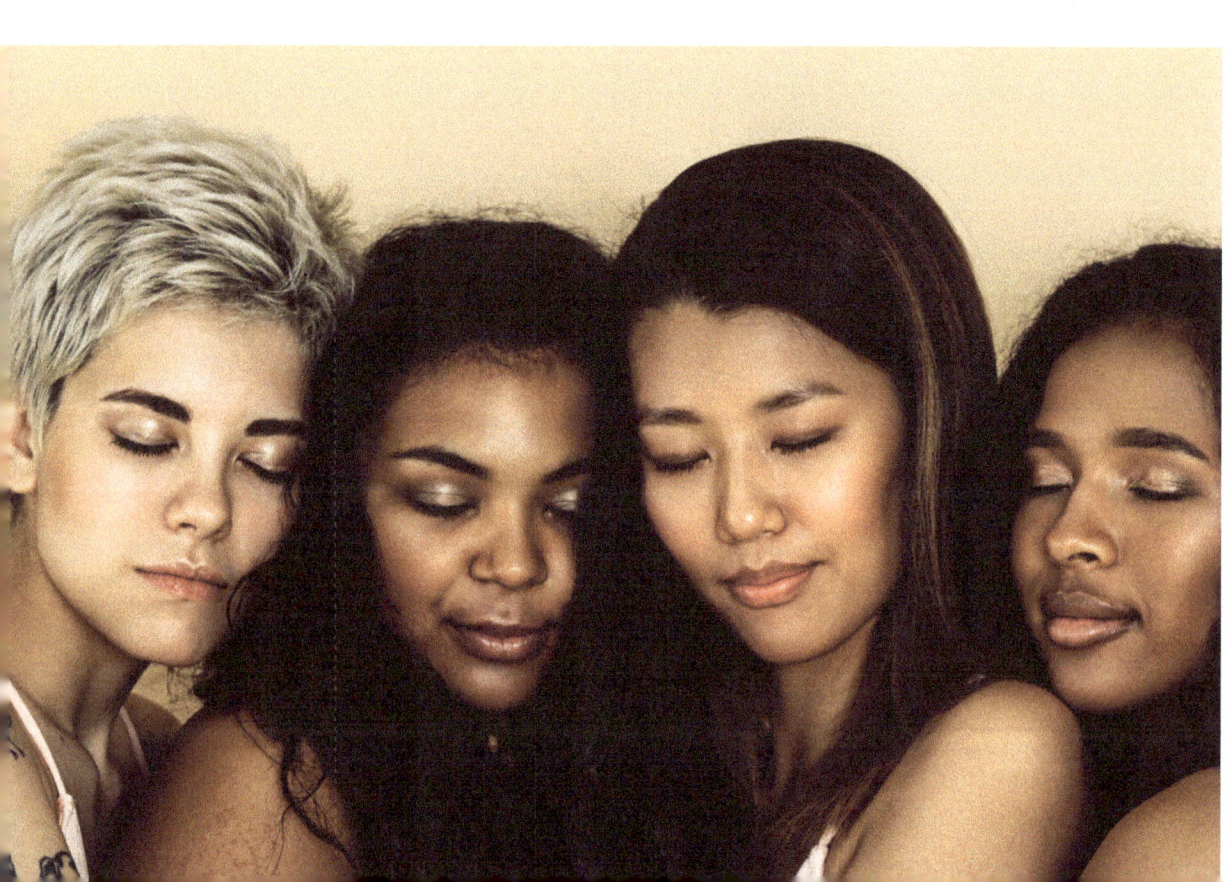

Healing is not meant to happen alone.

Whole-body support is based on the tools and systems you have set up around you, which does include other people, but it can also include a different mindset, environment, or way of being.

Every single person who has made it through depression, anxiety, autoimmune issues, or any other period of struggle will tell you without question that support is a basic requirement for making it to the other side. The birth of both a mother and baby is no different. Support isn't a luxury, it's essential to being healthy, happy, and whole.

Not all support is created equal. The support needed to heal in postpartum is not defined by the number of people in your life. More people does not always mean more support.

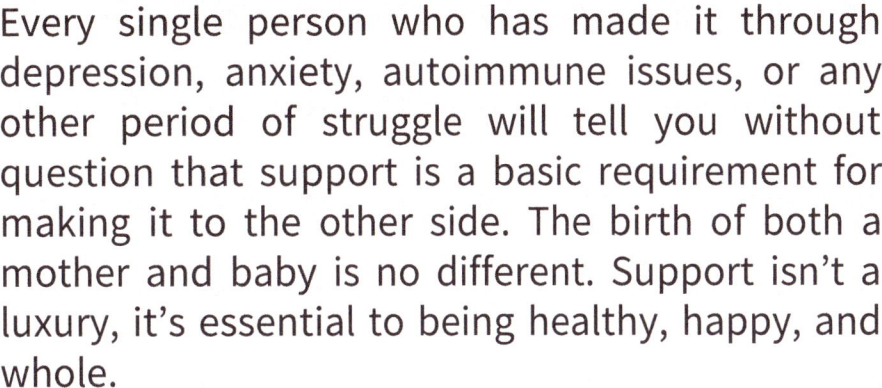

The key is to look at yourself - every piece - and determine what is needed in order for you to feel fully supported. Where are you struggling the most? In what ways do you need to lighten your load? This is a deeply personal process that will look different for everyone, and as mothers, we are often too busy to take the time to think this through, let alone take action. We are so busy co-regulating our children that we fail to put any care back towards ourselves. Our own nervous systems are begging for that level of attention and care.

In order to co-regulate in a way that feels good to you, there has to be space. This is where seeking out like-minded individuals that you feel strongly attuned and connected to provides immense value. There is a reason that the many generations before us honored the village and the community as a space where women came together to care for each other.

Our brains change dramatically when we are postpartum, and the reality is, we are wired to need support. It is necessary for proper nervous system regulation and function. Without it, none of us can truly thrive.

In the generations before us, these communities offered synchronous and consistent cycles of support in the postpartum months. Somebody was always around to help carve out the space needed for a mother and her new baby. This looked like everything from cooking meals to household chores to caring for the other children.

In our modern culture, this has shifted tremendously. We now carry this burden of insurmountable responsibility and societal pressure to the point where all women and families are feeling as if they have zero support (on top of feelings of failure, exhaustion, guilt, fear, etc.). Overwhelm has become the norm because we have so few support systems in place.

The bounce back culture that has been created over the last few generations is causing substantial harm to motherhood. And in order to end these feelings of mediocre motherhood and get back to feeling healthy and whole within our bodies, we must bring back the care and support we so desperately need.

Healing isn't linear

The path to healing is always paved with bends and twists and loops. Life happens, situations change, and there is always something new within yourself to discover and work through. Healing is much like a road without an end. Be gentle with yourself as you move through healing and know that your journey will ebb and flow right alongside life.

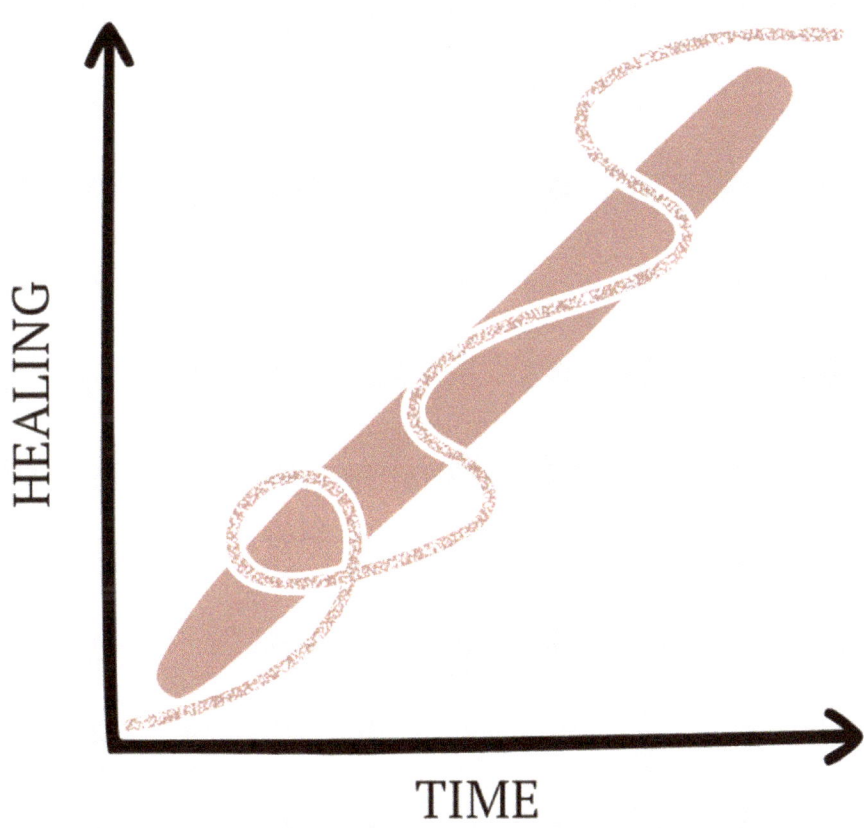

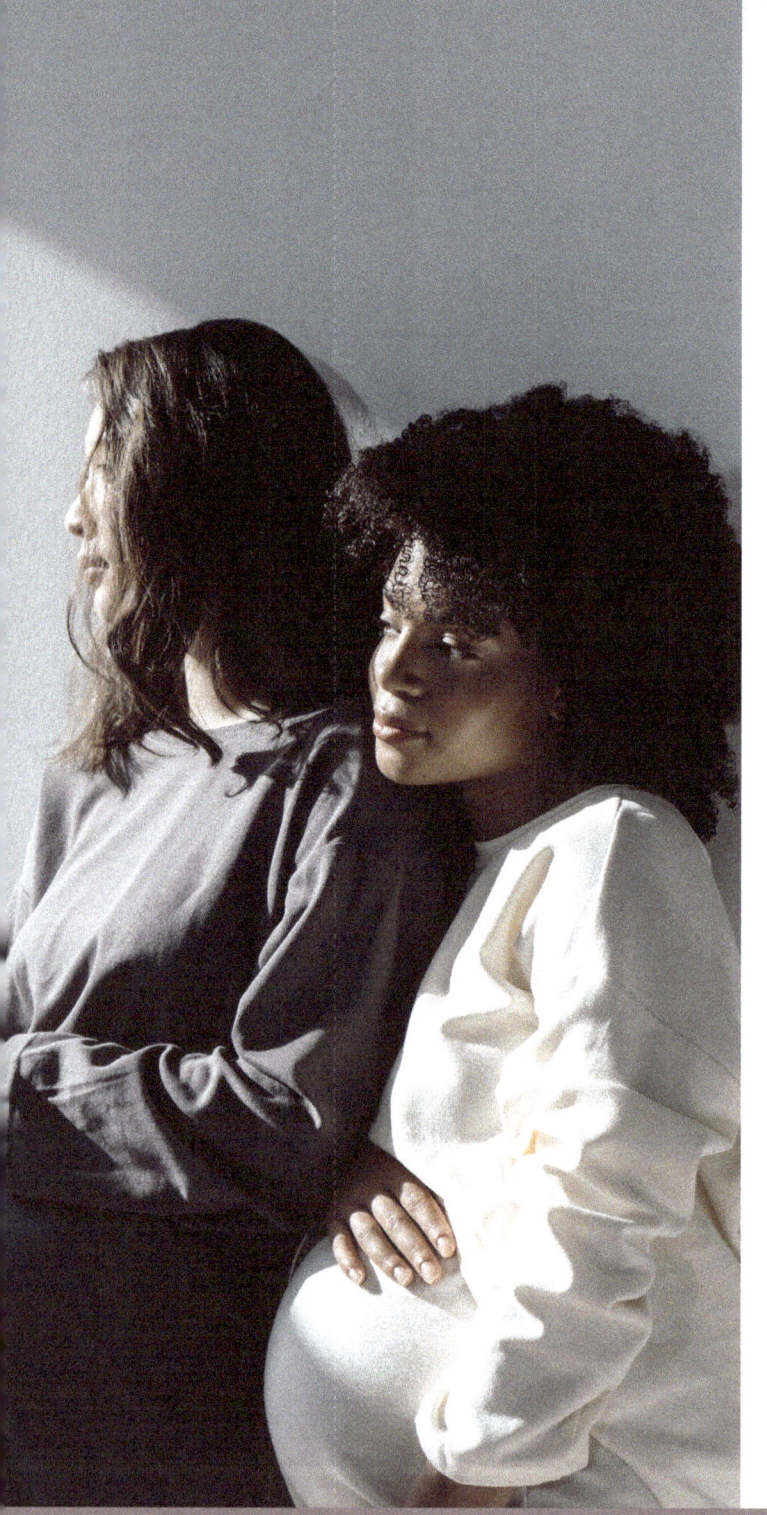

Steps to getting the right support

It starts with you.

Most women wait until the pain in their life is so significant that they have no other choice but to ask for help and seek out change. Then, when you finally decide that you are worth it, you are going to give yourself the time and attention to heal with clear boundaries, and you honor that, that is when things start feeling tricky.

That is when guilt starts creeping in and we start asking ourselves, "oh, is that okay? Can I do that?"

It is not okay for you not to have support. It is not okay for you to barely be surviving.

We are here to change the way women and mothers experience motherhood.

We are going to be moving you from the place you're in now to the place you deserve to be. But in order to do that, we have to get real and fully understand...Where are you now?

1. Assess where you are.

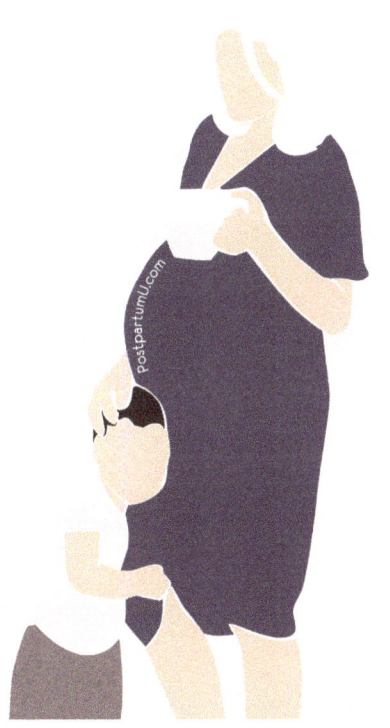

Taking an inventory of your physical, mental, emotional, and spiritual needs is essential to understanding what support you need in your life. In order to find the support you need, you have to get real and fully understand where are you now. When you understand where you are (your point A), you can better help yourself move to healing (your point B).

The first step to healing is taking the assessment to learn about your needs, keep track of your progress, and find exactly what you need to get better faster.

The Postpartum Recovery Assessment

Let's take a second to get clear about the state of your postpartum health. No matter where you are in your postpartum journey, this comprehensive assessment of your physical, mental, and emotional health, along with your health history, will be critical in removing the blocks to living your best life. You can take your free assessment at:

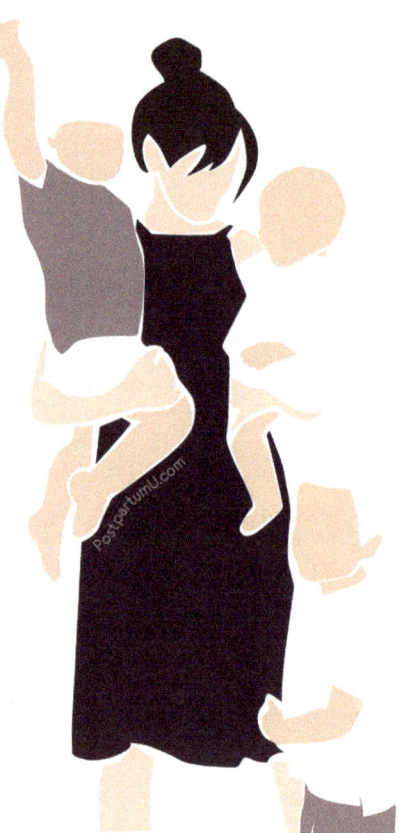

www.PostpartumU.com/Quiz

You can bring this assessment to your healthcare provider. If your provider hasn't asked you these questions or doesn't find it relevant, find a provider who will support you in whole-body healing. Use this to communicate with your partner about how you are feeling and come back often to reassess where you're at.

To heal, follow the principles outlined in this book and keep advocating for yourself until you find the support and answers you need to feel your best self again. You deserve nothing less.

Taking care of yourself is part of taking care of your children.

2. Find people to connect with.

Sisterhood and community are an absolute necessity on your healing journey. This will be a source of solace, celebration, knowledge, and self-discovery.

Reach out to your family and your community for support. Find professionals, groups, and others who can help you. Sometimes, it takes perseverance and creativity to find the right mix of support systems, depending on your personal needs and available resources.

I always encourage mamas to start in their local area. Find other mamas who need support and team up to care for each other's kids while you catch some down time. Or plan a meal exchange where everyone cooks one large meal for a few families and you swap, having a weeks' worth of nutritious meals already complete. Just these two ideas alone can ease a lot of the day-to-day stress of parenting!

If you don't have a local mama group, consider starting one. There are also many online options for getting one started and gathering people.

No matter what, don't stop until you find the care you need. If you aren't able to find the right provider, group, or support, keep looking. Don't stop reaching out and trying new support tools until you see the results you are seeking.

Creating Your Support Team

No matter where you are in your postpartum journey, having a team you can call on for support is an absolute must. Take a second to create your contact list. There is nothing more helpful than not having to think about who to call on in times you need it the most. Be sure to include names, numbers, and any important details.

Mom's Provider: _____

Baby's Provider: _____

Doula Support: _____

Breastfeeding Professional: _____

Counselor: _____

Chiropractor: _____

Local Mama Support Group: _____

Childcare/ Babysitter: _____

Housework: _____

Helpful Family/ Friends: _____

Download this worksheet here:

3. Constantly Reassess.

Always check with yourself. Ask, "What is it that I need in this moment?" "Where am I this week?" Life is always changing and requires re-evaluation so that you can continue healing and getting the right support you deserve.

Constantly reassessing is also critical because women often either discredit their healing completely or they belittle their own journey by minimizing, forgetting, or dismissing it ("oh, it wasn't that bad, I guess" or "you know, I didn't really do much, I just kept on pushing through..."). This takes away your own power by suppressing your intuition and autonomy.

Take time to review and reassess to meet your needs. Celebrate and rejoice in how far you come in your journey and always look at what you need in the short and long term. When you care for yourself, you simultaneously meet the needs of your family.

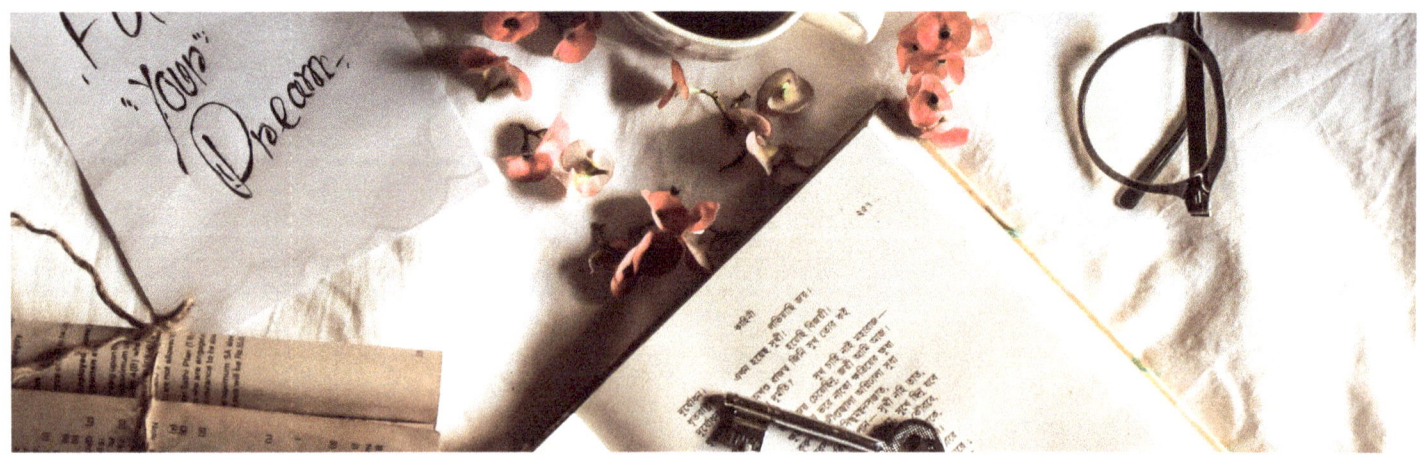

Personal Story: Amy C.

Amy C. had 2 amazing kids with the youngest being 2 years old. She had been a therapist for several years and knew she was skilled in the field but felt like she was missing something. She spent nearly her entire postpartum battling depression and no longer wanted to be on several medications for it. She also had a diagnosis of hypothyroidism, type 2 diabetes, and a long list of symptoms that felt beyond frustrating.

Amy knew her body wasn't broken, and she spent a great deal every month on supplements like probiotics, vitamin D, magnesium, B12, multi-vitamins, and many more. Although she didn't feel these supplements were doing anything great for her, she didn't feel like eating better was a good first step. However, she took my advice and started incorporating my recommendations into her day.

With each session, Amy would uncover major insights into her body, how she needed control to feel safe, her mom guilt and how that impacted her relationship with her children, her need to feel joy again, and so much more. Every time we dived in, there were new things that she was able to use and apply to her daily life and routine. She also started seeing how eating foods from the Postpartum Nutrition Plan took away many of her physical symptoms an gave her a great deal of energy. Along with the many tools listed in this book, Amy made some major lifestyle shifts that ultimately changed her life.

After working together for 5 months, Amy started losing weight. She was seeing her doctor again to reduce her medications altogether for both her depression and her hypothyroidism. Her relationship with both her husband and her two kids greatly improved. Even more, she felt so fueled by her new life that she de-cluttered and reorganized her entire home. Her renewed passion for life created the joy and health she had been missing for so long.

You can listen in to Amy's story in her own words (along with many other inspiring healing stories) on our website: www.PostpartumU.com/Testimonials

Personal Story: Mallory J.

At nearly 5 years postpartum, Mallory was still deep in the throes of postpartum depression and ill health. She had been on medication for her depression for 4 years and felt extreme fatigue, terrible acne, gut issues, low libido, resentment and anger toward her birth story, trouble connecting with her son, and barely hanging on in survival mode. She described getting out of bed in the morning as nearly an impossible feat, and she often crawled back in after getting her son ready for his day.

Mallory describes the process of working together: "Maranda transformed my health by giving me a meal plan, focusing on nutrition and gut health, and providing specific and unique ideas for me personally to do each day to heal my body. We worked on healing deep wounds, creating a new routine, and basically transforming every aspect of my life." By using the tools outlined in this book in order, we were able to make significant improvements in her health and well-being.

During our time together, as Mallory's symptoms improved, she worked alongside her doctor to reduce her depression medication. Within 5 months, she had completely weaned off medication and was symptom-free. No depression. No gut health issues or acne, the return of her libido, and even a desire to play with her son and experience a positive relationship.

To top it off, Mallory felt so confident in her new healthy body that she quit her job and begin working her dream job making double the income. "I literally went from surviving to thriving. I can honestly say Maranda helped me love life again. Through our healing and coaching sessions, she not only healed the physical but the emotional as well."

Personal Story: Olivia J.

Olivia came to me when her baby had just turned 19 months and she was so nervous for our initial consult, she was physically shaking. She spent months working with both a naturopathic provider and a therapist and felt minor improvements but didn't feel anywhere close to healing or feeling better. As she expressed to me, she was scared that she was out of options and that her marriage was coming to an end because of it.

During her postpartum months, Olivia felt intense anxiety, fear, depression, and even rage. She had intense outbursts towards her husband, and after blowing up at him for what she felt was the smallest things, she would cycle into guilt and depression. She knew that her marriage was on the brink of divorce but didn't feel she could stop the roller coaster.

To top it off, her anxiety caused panic attacks that left her afraid to even leave the house. Intrusive thoughts ruled her life and the simple act of getting dressed, answering the phone, or eating felt next to impossible. Because of this, Olivia began to experience autoimmune symptoms including bloating, food sensitivities, intense fatigue, and menstrual distress.

When we first started working together, we immediately started with nutrition and special herbal teas with the Postpartum Nutrition Plan. Because of her intense labor and history of anemia, Olivia began a liquid iron supplement along with a magnesium supplement for her nervous system. The effects were immediate and she started to notice more energy, no more bloating, and fewer mood swings.

As her energy increased, we were able to focus on establishing more balance in her nervous system and get her some powerful tools to help her in moments of anxiety. She incorporated art and journaling into her daily routine, along with breathing practices and more.

By month 3 (half way through the program), she no longer experienced any rage or outbursts towards her husband. Olivia's anxiety had ceased, she no longer had panic attacks, was getting out of bed in the morning with excitement, and even felt safe to start bringing her daughter to the park, where she started to meet new friends and build relationships with other moms.

By the end of our time together, Olivia was already speaking to other postpartum women and giving them tools to support them in their health and recovery. She not only felt she healed her body and marriage, she also found her life's passion helping other moms do the same.

You can listen in to Olivia's story in her own words (along with many other inspiring healing stories) on our website: www.PostpartumU.com/Testimonials

It takes strength.

It takes strength to raise our children. We are breaking these generational patterns that do not serve us so that when our children cross this threshold, they have the support that they need, and they have it without guilt or shame.

When you take care of your health and well-being and you set and honor boundaries, other people will listen.

I need to be able to spend 30 minutes in the shower alone.

I need to be able to journal at the end of my day.

I need to go on a walk by myself for 20 minutes so that I can take a breather.

I need to make sure that my kids are in bed at a certain time.

We have to lay these boundaries down and that is okay. It does not make you a bad parent. It does not mean that we are not meeting the needs of our family or our children.

If you are leaving your family to take time for yourself and feeling guilty the entire time, it is necessary to look deeper. Where is this coming from? Is this rooted in trauma? Is there a support system in place for you?

Back to the Roots

A Story from Around the World

In many parts of **Latin America**, the la cuarentena, meaning "quarantine", is a 40-day period of bonding with baby and healing the mother's body. During this time, she is not to work or perform any household duties, as doing so is believed to create exhaustion and mental challenges later in on in motherhood. She constantly receives check-ins from her midwife for the first several weeks, and is always served a homemade chicken soup. A mother's abdomen is usually wrapped in a cloth called a faja to help her keep her belly warm and to support her uterus in returning to its proper place. It's commonly believed that if the uterus is not in its place, nothing in her life will be in balance.

2. Nutrition

You'll learn:
- Common Misconceptions
- Maximizing Nutrient Intake
- Food as Medicine + Recipes
- Immune Boosting Herbs
- The Art of Supplementing

Chapter Two

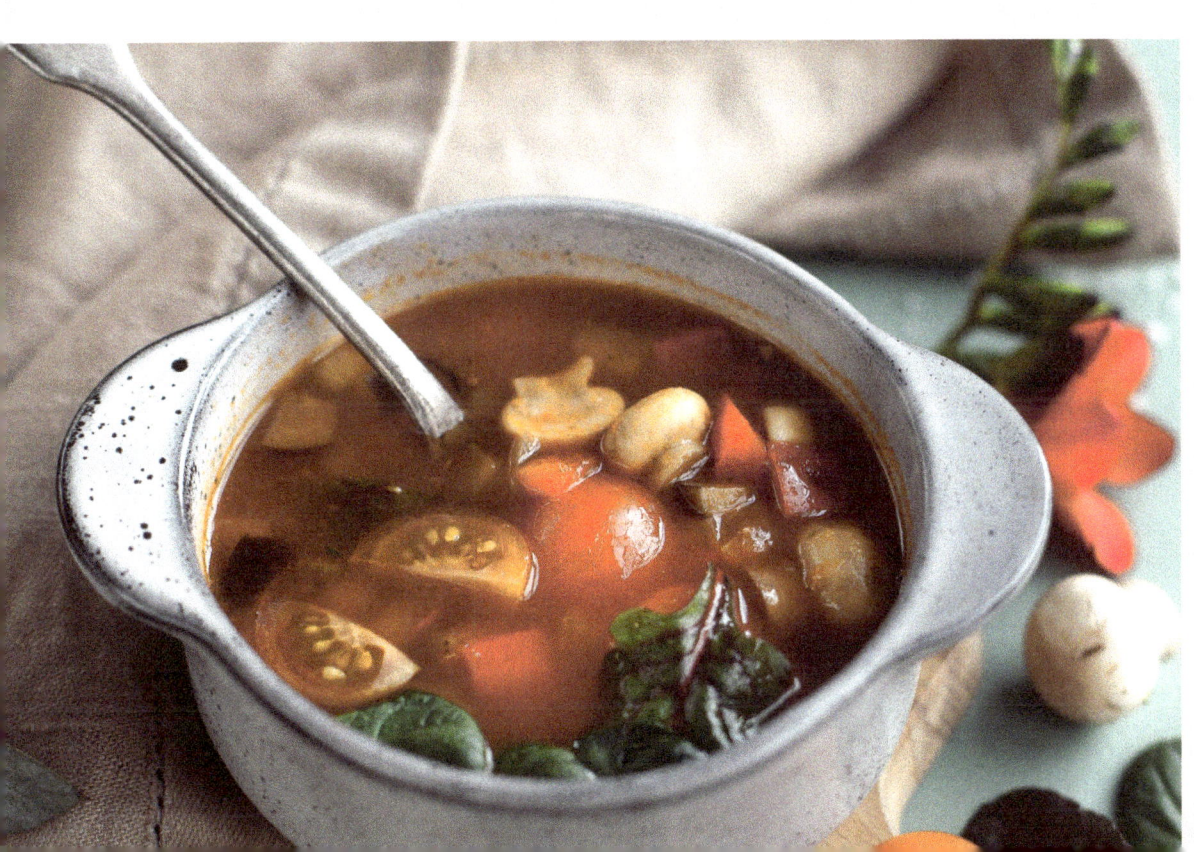

Nutrition is the foundation to health.

What you put into your body will become your body, so much so that the mark of dis-ease and mental health challenges are born in lack and deficiencies.

Every function and process in your body runs on the nourishment you provide it. In the months and years of recovery, repletion becomes paramount for healing, hormone balance, and overall wellness.

Study after study on postpartum depression and anxiety, as well as autoimmune disease and immune dysfunction, are finding that those who are deficient in key nutrients are also likely to have these major health issues.

Most mamas are deficient because:

1. The ability to absorb nutrients in postpartum decrease due to the physiological gut changes that occur after birth. A lack of enzymes and gastric acids make absorption a challenge. Without proper support, this can carry on for months or years. No matter how well you eat you don't absorb the nutrients, making you more deficient.
2. Growing a baby is hard work that takes a lot of nutrients from your body.
3. People have grown to rely on supplementation, which can have negative consequences.

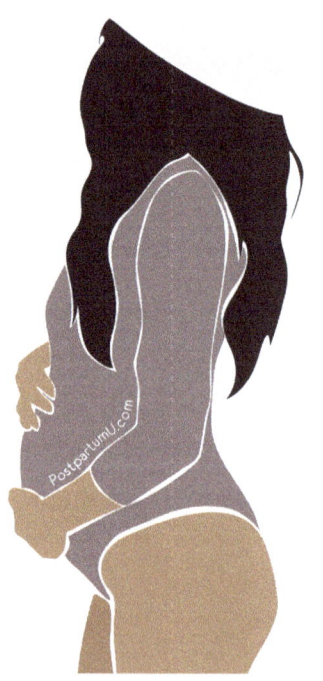

Our modern world has failed to understand how radically unique the postpartum body is. These unique physiological changes make postpartum nutrition counterintuitive to everything we hear about healthy food.

Common trends and ideas would have us believe that salads and smoothies would be ideal. However, these are some of the worst foods to consume when healing the body. Right along with casseroles, these food choices create challenges for digesting (one of the reasons gas, bloating, and stomach discomfort are so common).

What is healthy in postpartum is not based on just how nutrient-dense a particular meal is, but also how easy it is for the body to absorb. Not only do you need more nutrients to support healing, breastfeeding, and overall repletion from growing and birthing a baby, **you must consider and support the absorption of the nutrients you are consuming.**

This is one reason why supplementation isn't usually beneficial. If it's hard for the body to digest food because of its inability to absorb well, it certainly will have a hard time doing the same for a man-made pill; not to mention that most of these supplements on the market aren't regulated or vetted for quality.

For these reasons, it's best to stick with WHOLE FOODS that are easy to digest to maximize nutrient intake and to use supplements carefully, as I will further describe.

7 Powerful Postpartum Nourishing Principles

When eating in postpartum, it's important to follow a few basic nourishing principles that address your unique body changes. Doing so will ensure that you are absorbing the most nutrients from your foods (helping you feel better faster).

Follow these universal nourishing principles to create foods that heal your mind, body, and soul.

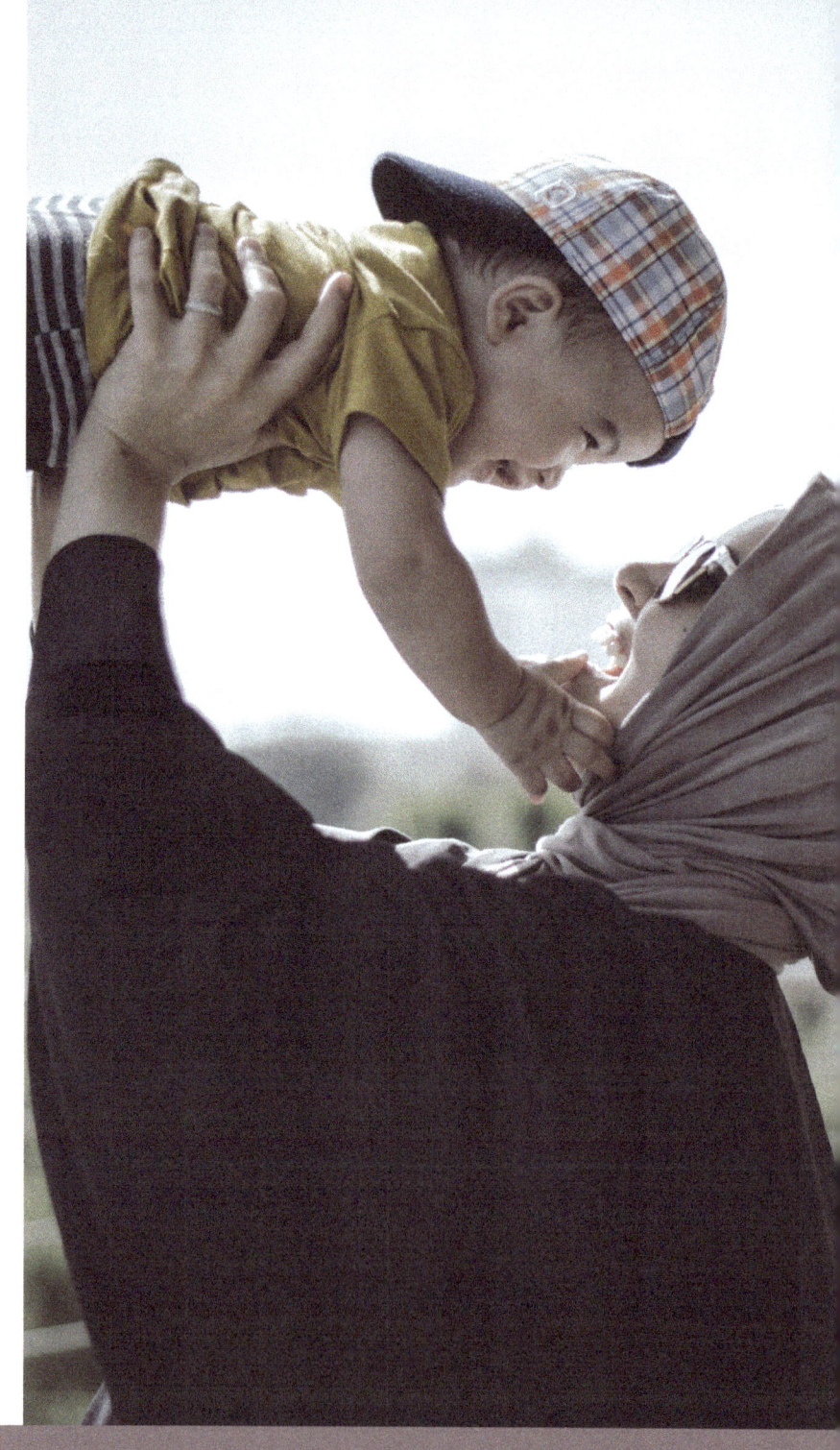

1. Eat warm foods.

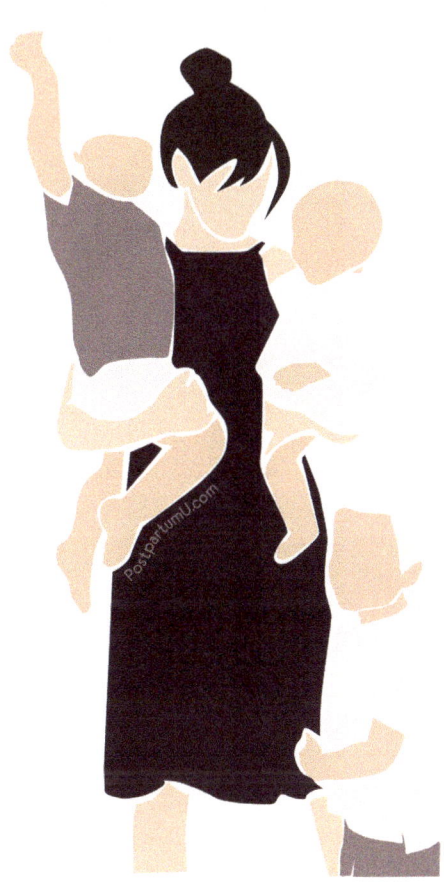

Eating foods that are warm can make a major difference in your healing alone. It sounds funny, but this worldwide cultural tradition is also clear in science. When we have a specific kind of injury (and for you, that means having given birth), heat and warmth are used to heal the body by providing proper blood circulation (critical for healing wounds). Warmth also allows for proper oxygenation, a necessary tool in combating harmful bacteria, and even supports regeneration of tissue within the uterus and perineum.

Cold foods and drinks contract blood vessels and makes it harder for the body to digest nutrients, especially fats (which are essential in postpartum for healing and your milk supply for baby). Even when a body isn't in postpartum, it will expend a great deal of energy warming up the consumed contents to an acceptable temperature within your body. Energy isn't something a postpartum body has a great deal of, and it's certainly not something you want to give away to warming whatever you have ingested.

2. Cook all fruits and veggies.

Your postpartum body lacks digestive enzymes, which are necessary for breaking up foods and supplying your body with nutrients needed for hormone balance and regulation, milk supply, and overall healing and health.

Due to the amount of energy necessary to break down foods, it's simply easier for the body to receive foods that are easy to digest. Cooking helps break down the nutrients for you so your body is able to get what it needs faster and without exerting any extra energy to get there.

3. Stay away from gluten and dairy

Gluten and dairy may not always seem like a nuisance for some, but studies are clear that they are a source of major inflammation. Inflammation is the foundation of dis-ease. Because the postpartum body is so sensitive, many struggle with both. The proteins of both gluten and dairy stay in the body for six weeks, so it's best to eliminate these foods for six weeks or longer to see results.

4. Eat meals rich in protein and fats.

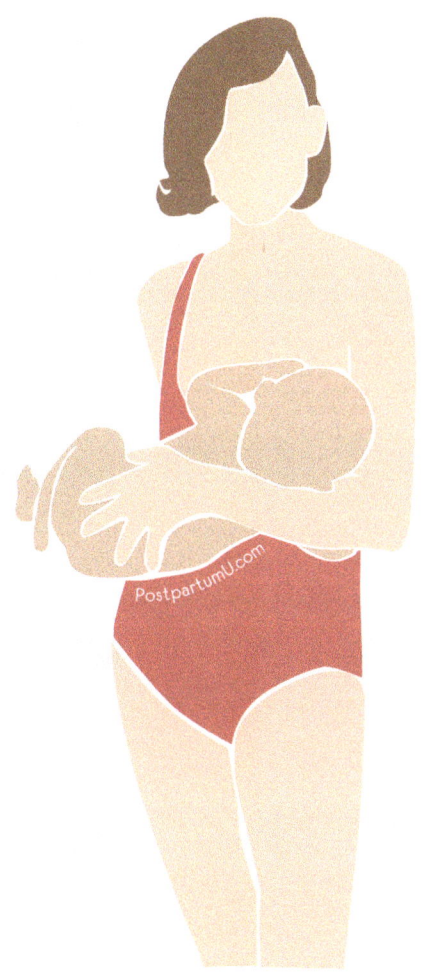

Eating a high protein and fat diet is essential to healing after birth. Protein is the building block in which your cells are made, and fats are required for hormone regulation, milk production, and tissue repair. Be sure to consume plenty, particularly from animal products.

Animal products are some of the most nutrient dense bio-available foods on the planet. Most cultures around the world that practice veganism or vegetarianism will forego these practices during postpartum because of their necessary healing properties derived nowhere else.

5. Be mindful of your food and how you feel.

We all know that many foods are considered comforts. The term "comfort foods" has existed for ages. Food does have an impact on the way we feel, both good and bad, especially in postpartum. As you eat, pay close attention to how your body feels with food. Use what you learn to your advantage.

For example, if eating chicken soup made you feel less anxious, eat it the next time you feel that way. Or if you notice that every time you consume eggs you get indigestion or fatigue, you may have a food sensitivity or allergy. Even if it's deemed a healthy food, your body can react negatively to it. Listen in and honor your body accordingly.

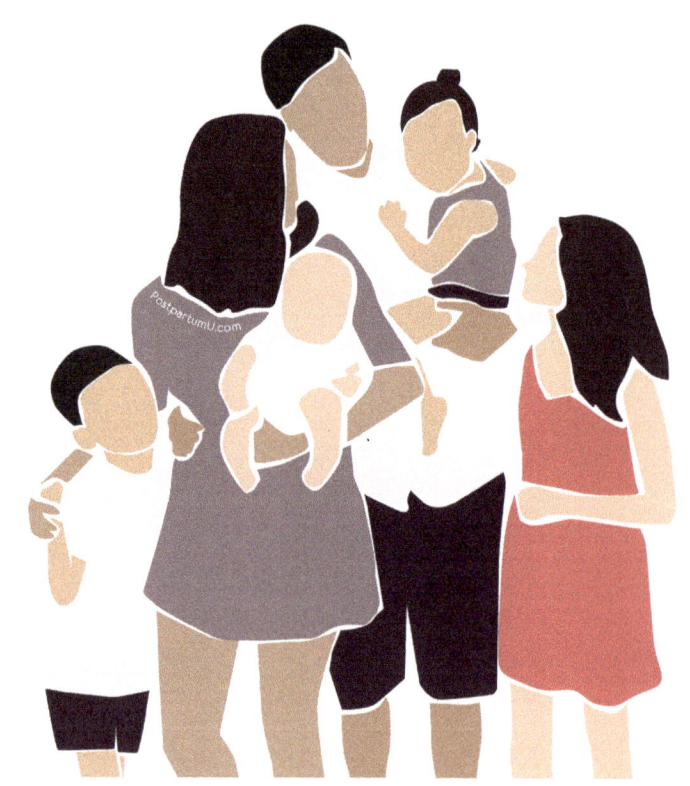

6. The simpler the better.

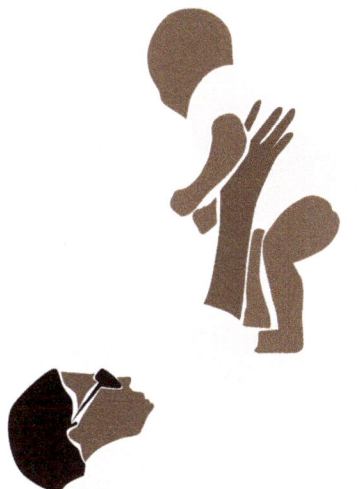

As Michael Pollen says, "Eat food; not too much, mostly plants." No better advice could be given. Keep your recipes and meals simple. The more complicated the recipes, including hard to find or man-made ingredients, the harder it'll be for you to digest. Keep things simple.

7. Eat organic and local as much as possible.

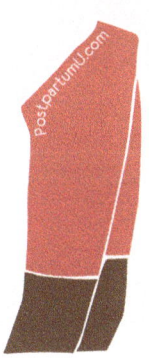

Eating organic means you steer clear of harmful hormones and pesticides in your food. Local means your food is fresher and more nutrient dense. It's okay if not all of your food meets these criteria, but whenever possible, know that it's worth the investment.

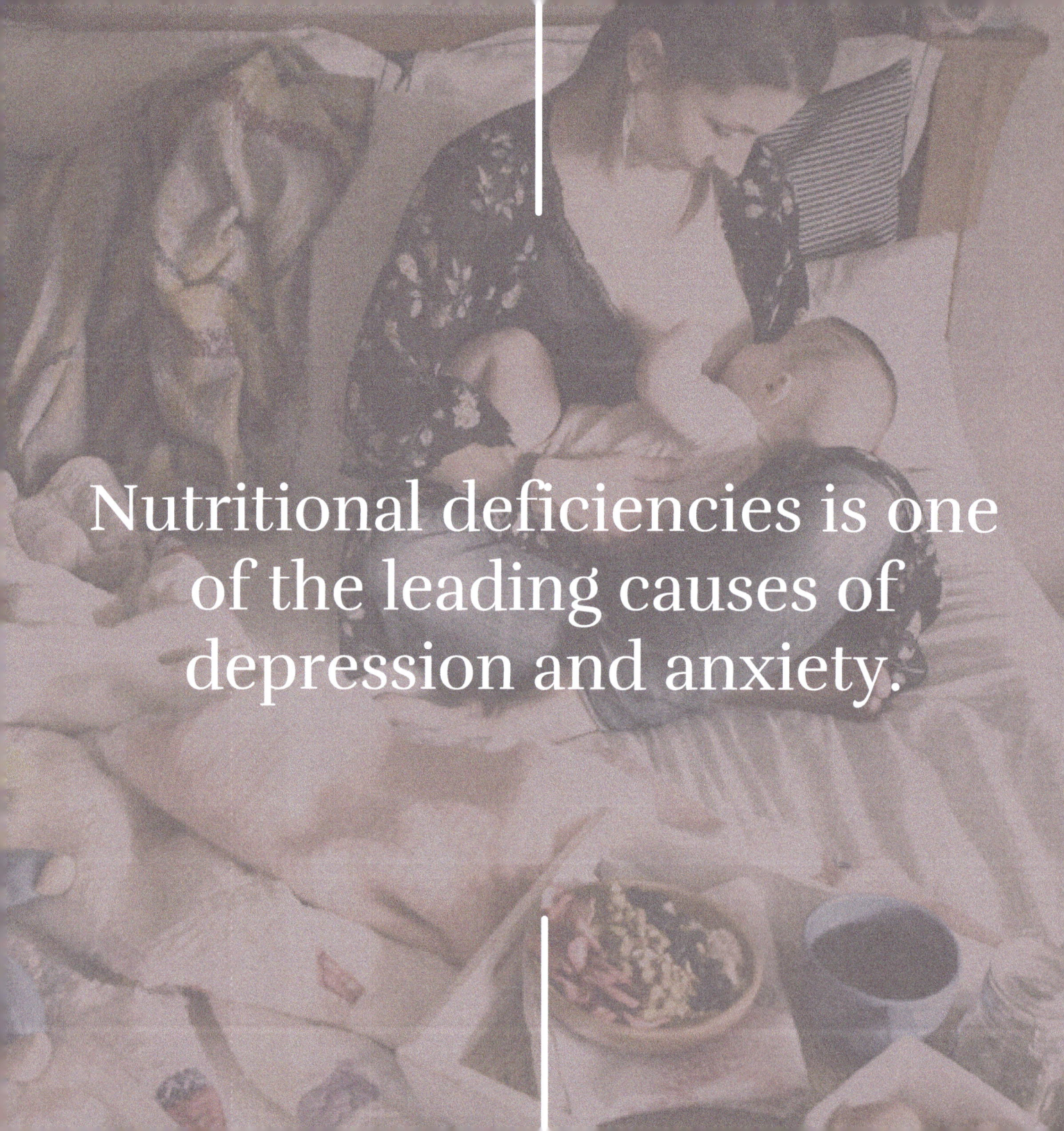

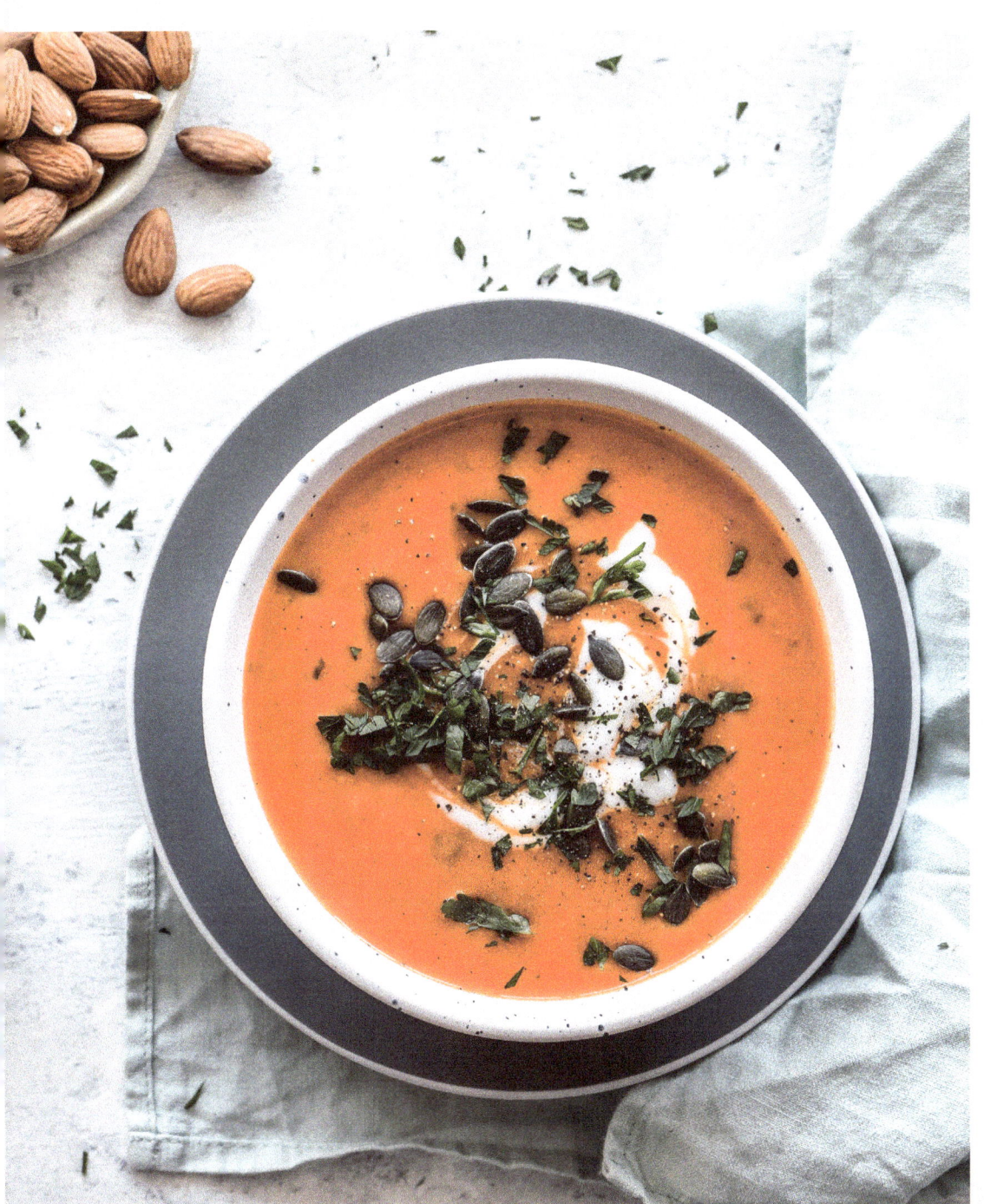

Food as Medicine + Recipes

Recovery Soup

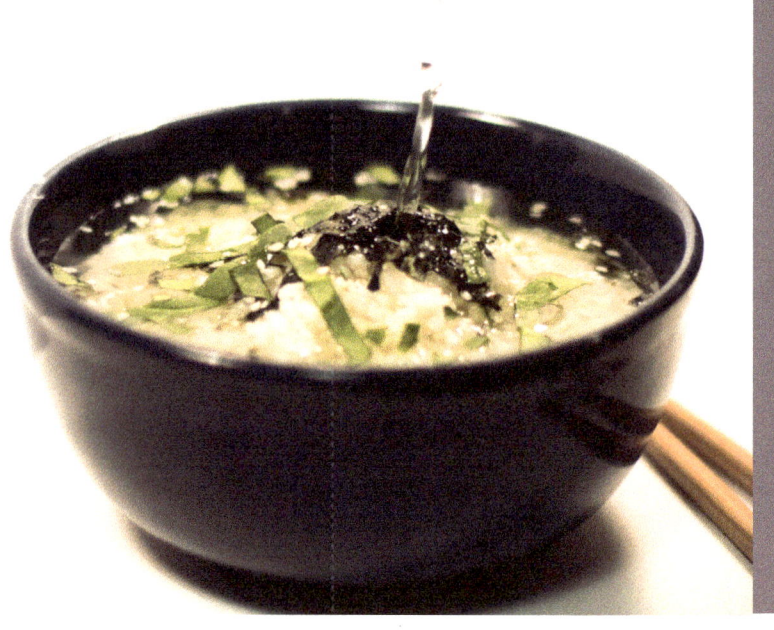

From the Postpartum Nutrition Plan

Ingredients:

- 3 tablespoons butter
- 1 medium chopped onion
- 3 chopped carrots
- 2 chopped leeks
- 3 medium potatoes cubed
- 3 large tomatoes cut/cubed
- 1 cup rinsed quinoa
- 8 cups beef broth
- .5 squeezed lemon
- 1 teaspoon turmeric
- .5 teaspoon sea salt
- .5 teaspoon black pepper
- 1 tablespoon of ground cumin

Instructions:

1. Sauté the onions, leeks, and carrots in butter until tender.
2. Place all ingredients in a large pot. Bring to a boil then reduce to a low simmer for 30 minutes. Stir occasionally and be sure your veggies are tender.
3. Serve hot or let cool before placing in freezer bags or mason jars.

Bone Broth

From the Postpartum Nutrition Plan

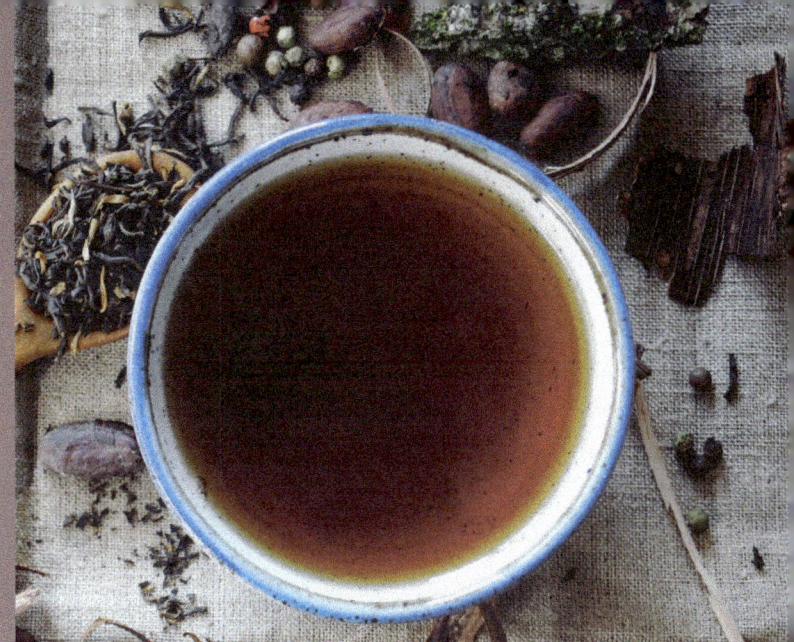

Ingredients:

- 2.5 pounds beef soup bones
- 2.5 pounds beef marrow bones
- 8 cups water
- Shot apple cider vinegar
- Handful carrots
- Handful celery stocks
- 1 coarsely chopped onion
- 2 tablespoons parsley
- 2 tablespoons sea salt
- 2 teaspoons black pepper

Instructions:

1. Roast all bones in oven for 30 minutes. Once done, place all ingredients in a crockpot for 24 hours, adding water as necessary. You can also cook all in an Instant Pot for 120 minutes.
2. Strain the broth, being sure to squeeze the juice out of the vegetables.
3. Let cool before placing in freezer bags or mason jars.

DO NOT DISCARD THE GELATIN THAT FORMS ON THE TOP.

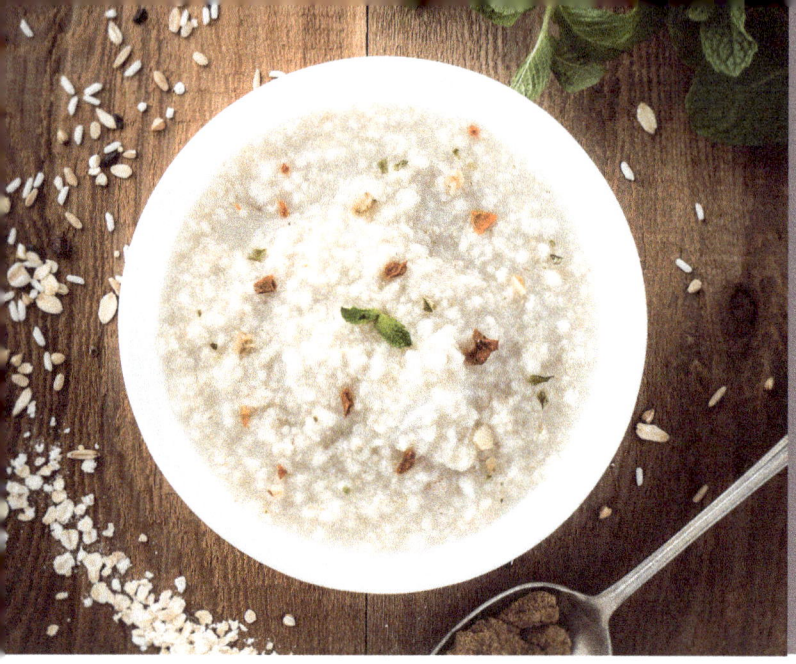

Oatmeal Porridge

From the Postpartum Nutrition Plan

Ingredients:

- 3 half pint mason jars
- 1 1/2 cup old fashioned oats
- 1/4 teaspoon chia seeds
- 1 cup water and/or milk alternative per jar
- add raspberries before serving

Instructions:

1. Fill each jar with ½ cup of dry old-fashioned oats and a generous sprinkle of dry chia seeds. Store away until ready to use.
2. The night before the intended use, add 1 cup of water and/or milk alternative to the jar, put the lid back on, and place it in the fridge to soak the oatmeal.
3. Before serving, warm the contents of the jar and add berries.

Coconut Energy Balls

From the Postpartum Nutrition Plan

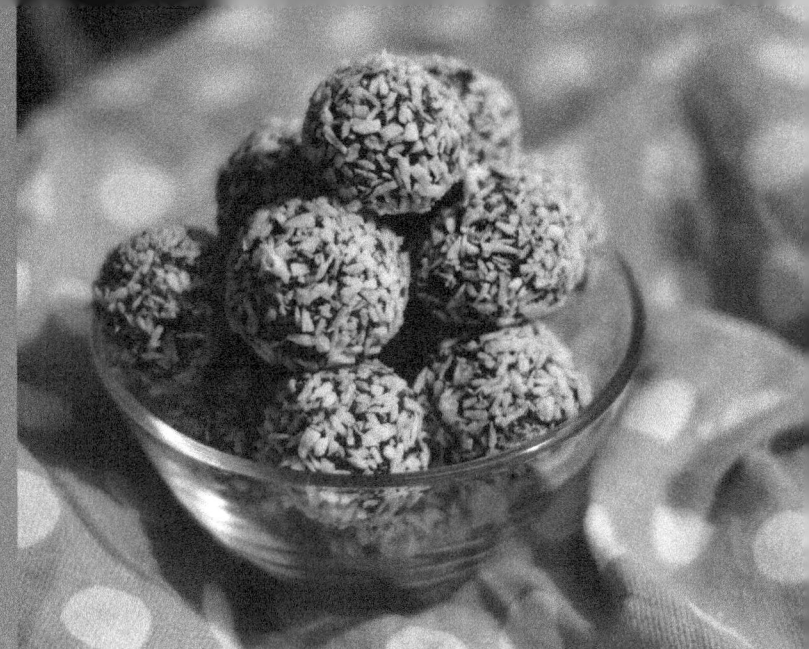

Ingredients:

- 1 cup pitted dates
- 3 tablespoons nut butter
- 1 tablespoon chia seeds, soaked overnight
- 2/3 cup old fashioned rolled oats, soaked overnight
- 1/4 cup chocolate chips
- 2/3 cup shredded coconut

Instructions:

1. In a food processor, pulse dates. Add in other ingredients except coconut.

2. Roll batter into balls and sprinkle with coconut.

3. Place in fridge for at least 15 minutes before serving fresh.

These are freezer safe so you can make a large batch for easy snacking.

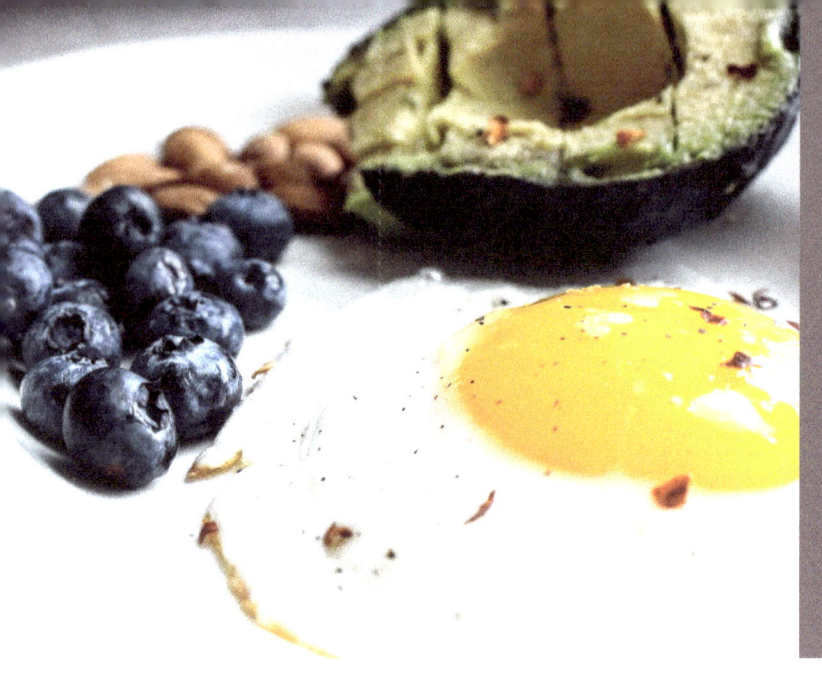

Snacks List

From the Postpartum Nutrition Plan

- Mixed nuts roasted in oil or fat
- Pan fried avocado with bacon
- Scrambled eggs
- Egg muffins
- Hard boiled eggs
- Deviled eggs
- Sweet potato with olive oil, chives, and spices
- Coconut energy balls
- Warm papaya
- Warm fresh berries
- Lactation cookies
- Coconut and fig with roasted granola
- Bean and rice gluten free burrito
- Fried rice
- Oatmeal with berries and chia seeds
- Avocado toast
- Warm applesauce
- Roasted chickpeas

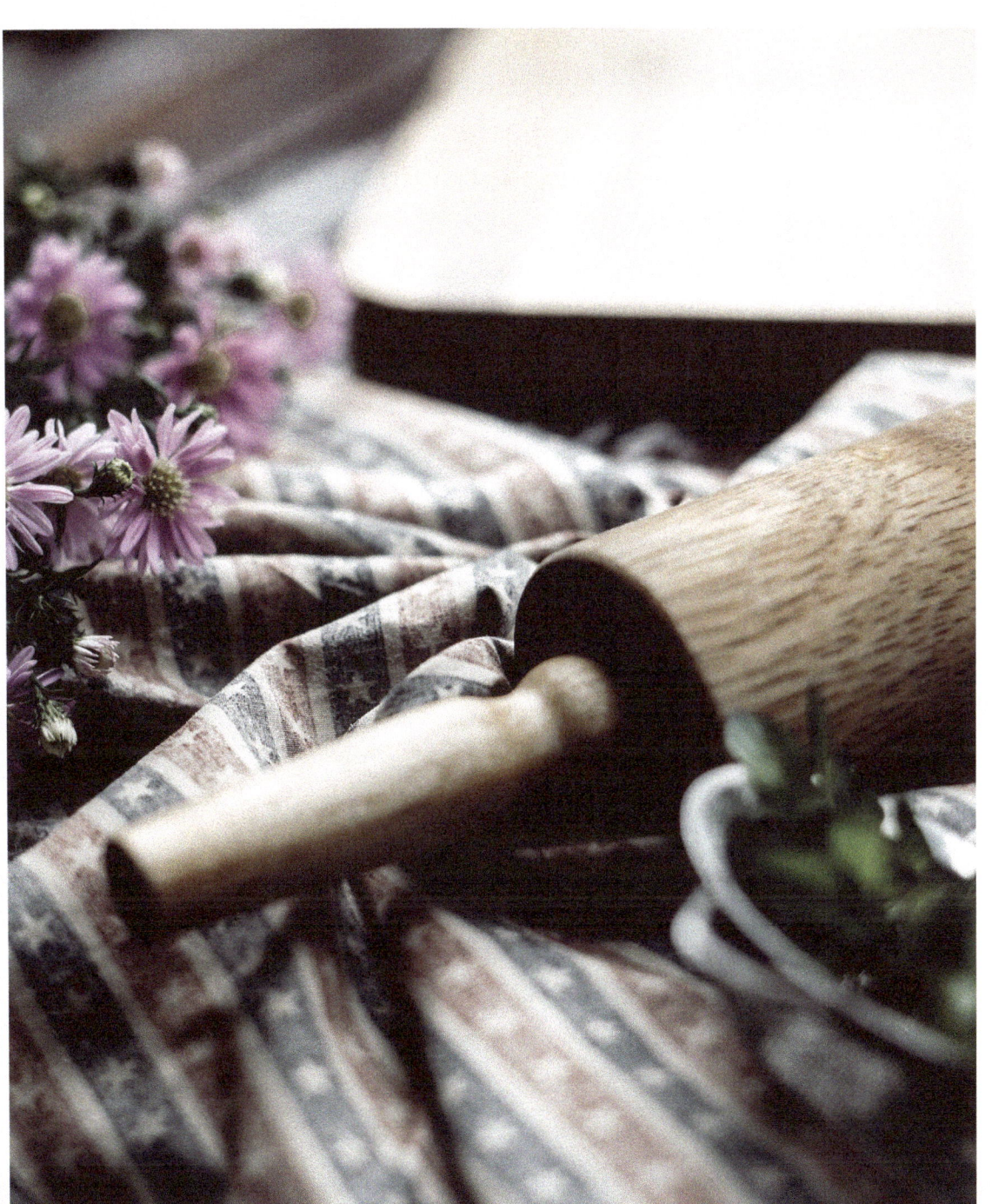

Herbs and Supplements

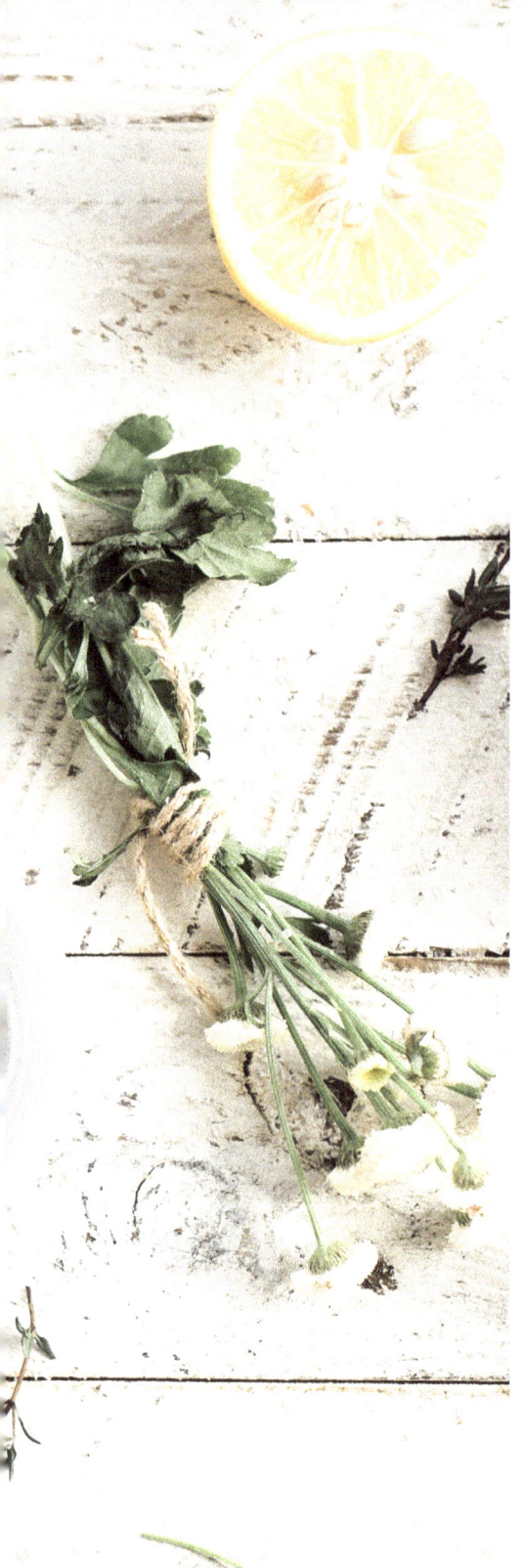

Healing Postpartum Herbs

Herbal teas and tinctures are by far a favorite way to get nutrients packed into a small serving. Drinking many of your nutrient requirements in one glass of tea is one of the most invigorating energy boosts and one of my clients' favorite parts of healing.

Herbs are nothing to fear. Over the last few decades, the healthcare industry and medical market has successfully placed fear, worry, and anxiety over herbs, marking them as dangerous, unknown, and highly risky, especially in pregnancy and postpartum. It's best to always do your research and connect with your local herbalist if you feel unsure.

I am recommending herbs that are as simple and nutrient-dense as can be. The nutrients within them contain properties that are essential to healing the body. They are packed with goodness, support immune system, and are amazing for building back the nutrient stores of postpartum women. All of these are safe for breastfeeding and pregnancy, unless otherwise mentioned.

Stinging Nettle

This is not only an herb that reduces stress and tension, but it's also prized for its anti-inflammatory properties. It's high in easily digestible iron, calcium, and folic acid. Its benefits go well beyond this guide.

Oat Straw

This herb is known for its ability to support mamas in creating more milk when breastfeeding. It's high in calcium and magnesium and reduces tension and stress.

Echinacea

Echinacea is powerful herb full of antioxidants that reduces inflammation, boosts the immune system, and is even known to be a cancer killing machine. Only use this when you feel illness coming, rather than a constant preventative herb.

Calendula

This is an anti-viral herb full of Vitamin C and Vitamin E. It targets symptoms of illnesses related to colds and has a history of use for smallpox and measles. This fever reducer and decongestant also supports elimination of menstrual cramps and pain. Do not use in pregnancy.

The Art of Supplements

There are few supplements that most women are in particular need of in addition to whole foods, especially in the years after childbirth. Some of these additional supplements include:

- Vitamin D
- Magnesium
- General Multivitamin
- Omega 3s
- Probiotics
- Iron
- Vitamin C and Zinc for immunity

If you choose to supplement, find brands that are not in your local supermarket. Stick to liquid or powder forms that will support better absorption.

Stay away from anything that contains folic acid, as you want to consume the natural version, folate. Avoid multivitamins with iron as it prevents absorption of other key nutrients. If you need an iron supplement, opt for a liquid that's taken separately from your multivitamin.

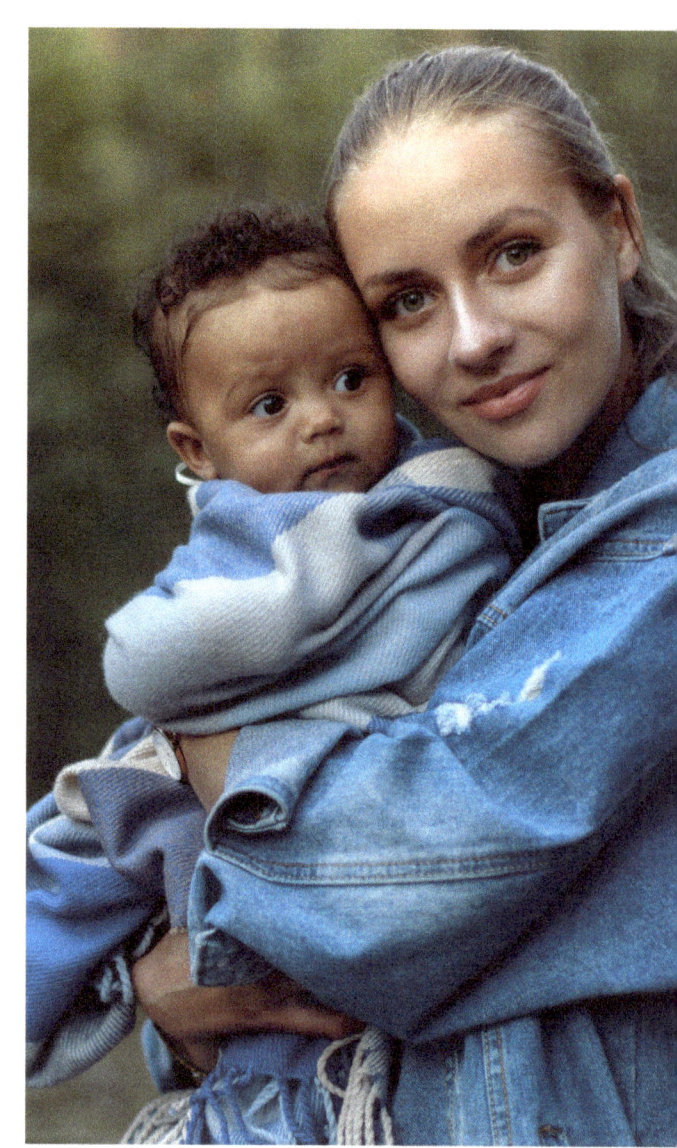

In addition, Vitamin D is a necessary for anyone who doesn't live near the equator. Look up your area's Vitamin D recommendations and supplement accordingly.

Many mamas like to take additional supplements of Omega 3s. Cod liver oil is great for getting more than just omegas (such as Vitamin A and D). However, fish oil tends to be richer in EPA and DHA. Both are great options and should be considered if you are not able to consume two servings of fish per week.

In terms of magnesium, the body does a much better job of absorbing it through the skin. Consider taking magnesium salt baths or foot soaks at least once a week rather than taking it in pill form. You can take Magnesium Calcite in powder form for additional support.

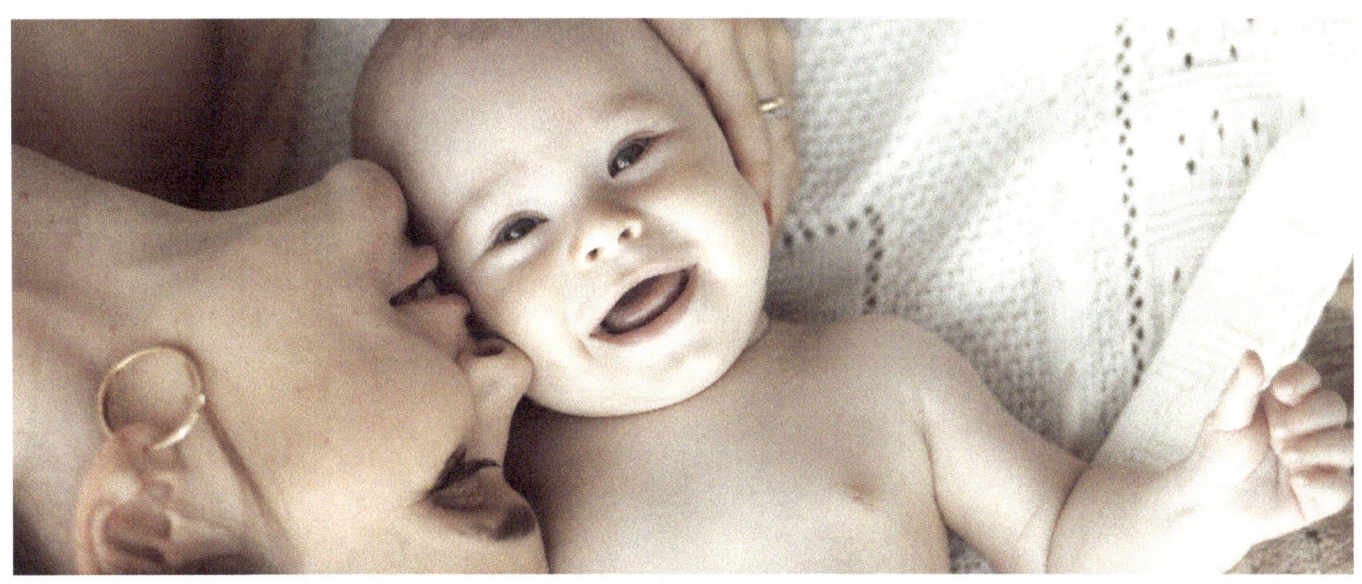

Back to the Roots

A Story from Around the World

Native American culture places a heavy affinity on ceremony. Everything is a ritual and celebration. A new mother is pampered and given ample time to rest and recover after the birth. She is bathed in a ritual involving warmth and herbs, and is placed in a sweat lodge to increase her circulation and release any toxins that have stored in her body during the pregnancy. Ceremonial foods are given to her in many stages by the elders of the community, welcoming her into motherhood. Alaska Native Americans believe that birth itself is a ceremony. The aunties, sisters, and mothers provide ongoing care, ensuring a mother and baby are gifted their ceremonial rites of passage.

3. Sleep

You'll learn:

- The Significance of Sleep
- Sleep to Heal
- Getting the Best
- Sleep Support

Chapter Three

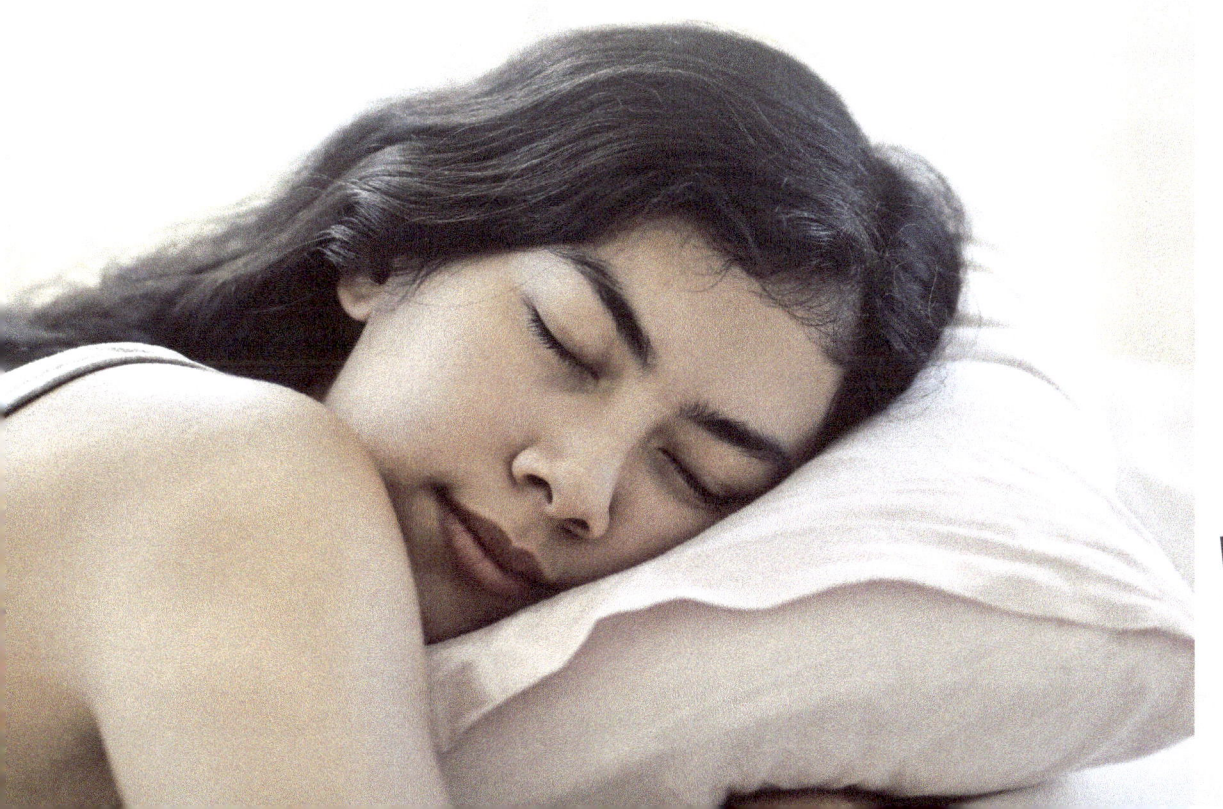

Getting sleep in the postpartum period is a multi-billion-dollar industry.

It seems like everyone has some technique or idea about how you should sleep.

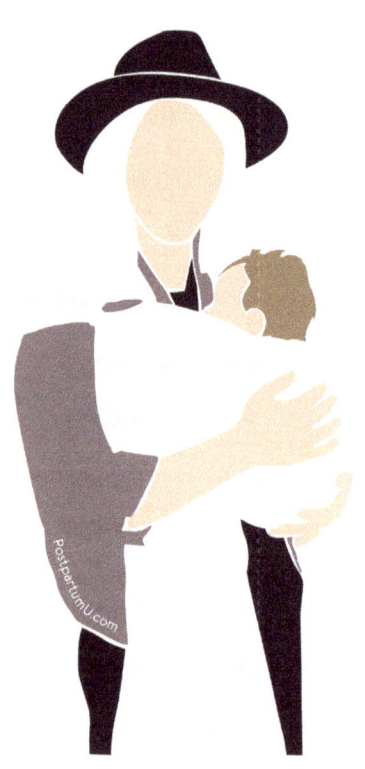

Sleep is essential for wellness, nervous system function, and immune health. No amount of self-care can replace your need for solid, deep sleep.

Much like nutrition looks different in postpartum, so too does quality sleep, and for much more obvious reasons.

However, there are other factors at play that are far less obvious when it comes to the physiological and mental changes that take place in postpartum. These greatly impact how quickly you fall sleep, how deeply you sleep, your REM cycle, and even how you wake up.

We ALL know and expect to have a baby that wakes often to nurse and be cared for. The fact is, your baby is biologically set to wake very often. It's a SURVIVAL technique that keeps your baby growing and alive, especially as they navigate living outside the womb.

You also help shape your baby's sleeping patterns by the way you connect with your child physically, emotionally, and energetically, as well as the way you HEAL your own postpartum body in the years following childbirth.

- How you connect with your baby alters their genetic patterns.
- How you mentally process your birth experience helps dictate how quickly you fall asleep, how much REM you get, and how well-rested you feel.
- What you eat is directly channeled to your hormones (which dramatically impact sleep, milk production, and your baby's resting patterns).
- Stress or feelings of depression and anxiety trigger the stress response in your baby, which creates a fussy baby who's more wakeful and sleep-deprived (creating a nasty dark spiral).

A postpartum body is designed to wake often.

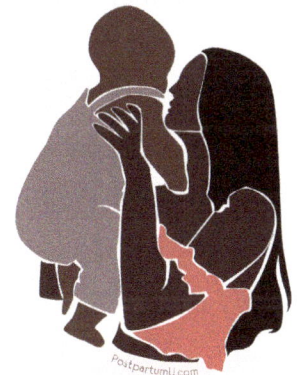

Getting the best sleep possible for yourself, as well as meeting your baby's needs, is doable…

…without sleep training your baby. As a matter of fact, it's more about sleep training parents than it is the baby.

It's important to note that your body is designed to wake often. Due to the chemical brain changes that have taken place after birth, you are now designed to fall asleep faster, rest more deeply, and to do so in smaller time frames. You are also biologically set to wake up more easily at the sound of your baby, or even to anticipate your baby's needs.

However, nutrient deficiencies, hormone imbalances, trauma, and severe exhaustion only make sleep feel that much more challenging. This is why incorporating several of the strategies in this guide is necessary to getting the most out of it. When you get the nutrients you need, your hormones get what they need to function better, which produces the hormones necessary to sleep deeper and faster. This then supports you in having more energy to cook foods that get you more nutrients…and the upward spiral continues.

And now that your body is getting the nutrients it so desperately needs, we can focus on getting you more sleep.

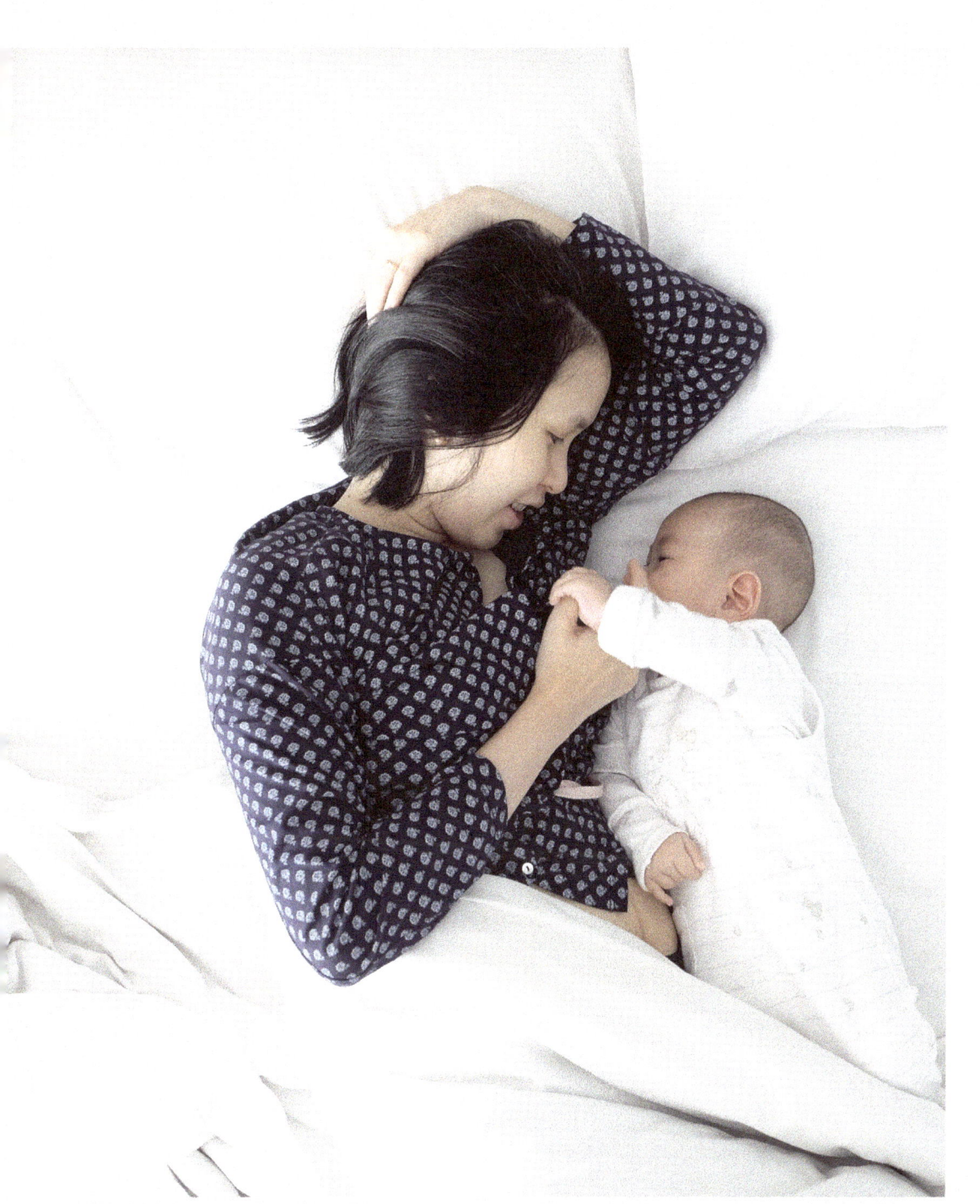

Creating and Planning for Better Sleep

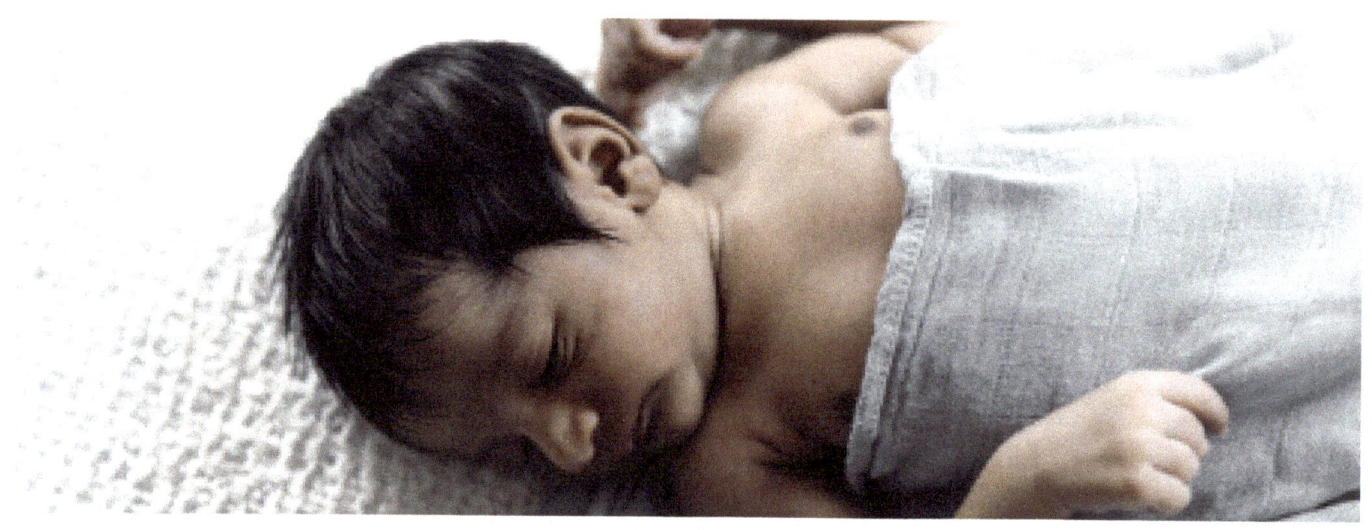

A Step-By-Step Better Sleep Plan

Many mamas wake up often in the middle of the night to breastfeed, pump, and/or care for their baby. As babies grow, they are able to sleep for longer periods of time without middle-of-the-night needs. It's important to find strategies that will allow your child to still get care without compromising your own needs.

You must first realize that deep quality sleep is possible even while you are waking frequently. To do this, though, means making sleep the absolute number one priority for your health and healing.

Now we're going to get you a personalized strategy to getting the best sleep while still giving your baby their care they need.

Your Sleep Plan:

Write your answers in the space provided.

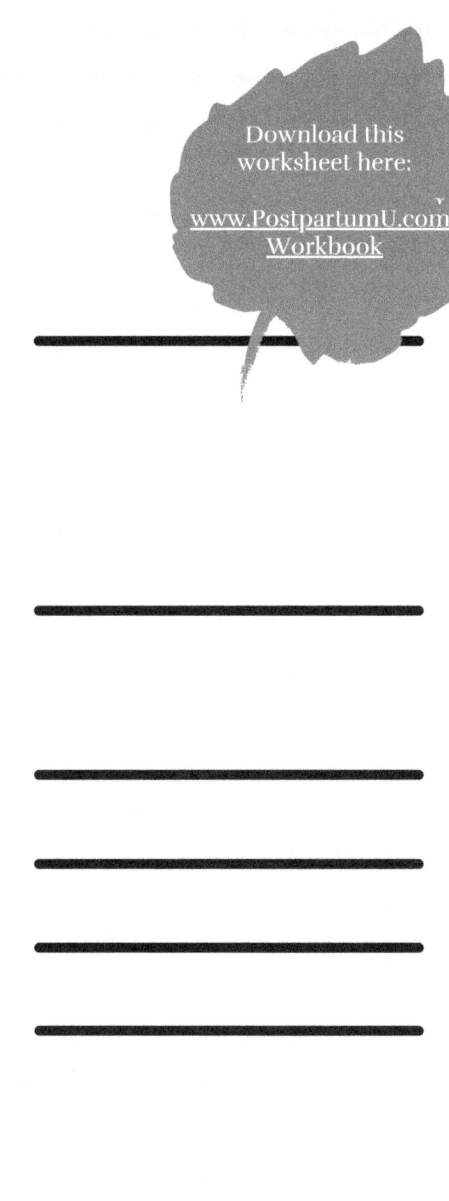

Download this worksheet here:
www.PostpartumU.com/Workbook

1. Calculate how many hours of sleep you need per night to feel rested and rejuvenated. Most women need about 9-12 hours of sleep per night when healing in the years after childbirth.

_____

2. Calculate how many hours you are awake in the middle of the night on average.

_____

3. Take a minute to assess if there are any ways in which you can minimize those hours. For example, bringing baby to co-sleep with you or in a bassinet next to you to limit the time you are out of bed. Prepare bottles before bed. Enlist your partner to take over from bedtime to 1AM. Get creative to see what's possible for you.

_____

_____

_____

_____

4. Adjust the number of hours you are awake in the middle of the night to accommodate those changes. Estimating is completely fine.

_____

Your Sleep Plan:
Write your answers in the space provided.

5. Add those wakeful hours to the number of hours of sleep you need per night. For example, if you are awake 3 hours a night, and your partner has agreed to watch baby until 1AM, by cutting off at least an hour of your time you can expect to wake 2 hours. Add 2 hours of sleep to your needed 9 hours for a total of 11 hours of sleep.

6. Determine what time you need to be in bed to support your needed hours of sleep based on the time you know you need to wake.

7. Make this bedtime your absolute number one priority. Try it. Adjust as you go. Keep an open dialogue with your partner about it. The more they see it is a priority for you, the more they will support you in your sleep and making sure you are getting enough.

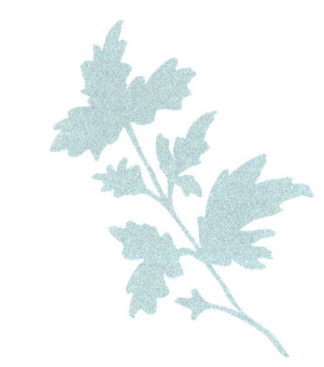

Back to the Roots

A Story from Around the World

Postpartum traditions in **India** include one of the longest periods of rest and rejuvenation, lasting between 40-60 days. Keeping the postpartum body warm is of utmost importance during this time. To do this, a mother's diet must include only nutrient-dense, easily digestible foods that are warming to the body. Massages are given daily with special oil blends and herbs to keep her blood circulation going, which aids in faster recovery. It's believed that providing warmth within and throughout the body consistently will create a stronger mother for life.

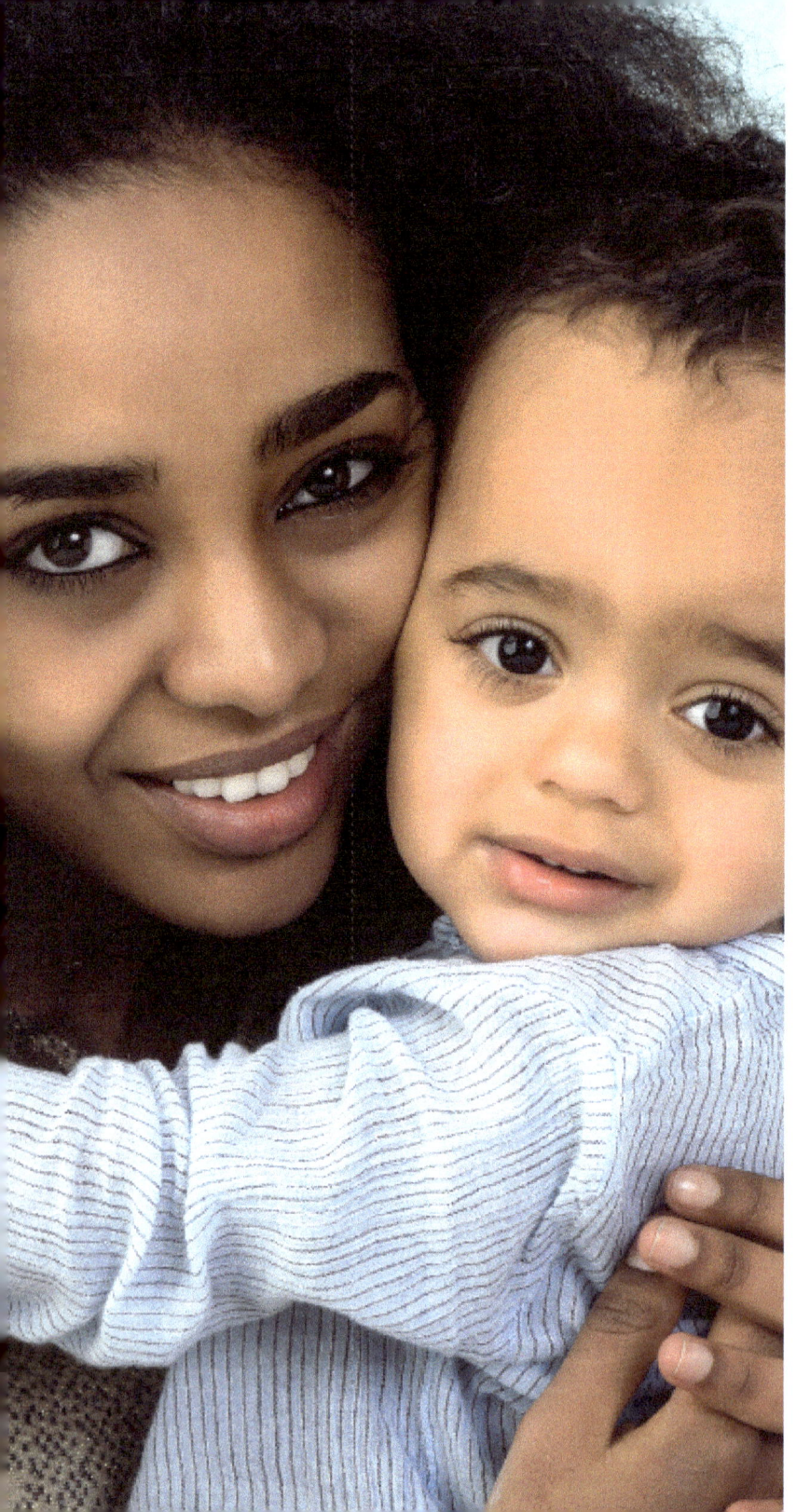

Extra Sleep Support

Routine

Set yourself and your family up for sleep success by creating a calming bedtime routine. Baths, lavender oil massage, a bedtime story...these are things you can do for yourself too, not just your baby/children.

Bedtime Tea

Honey chamomile, valerian root, or lavender tea makes for a great warming, relaxing, and sleep-inducing bedtime ritual. Couple this with 20 minutes of journaling and you have yourself the ultimate relaxation practice.

Humming

Close your eyes and mouth, hold your ears, take a deep breath, and hum for as long as you can. Do this for at least 5 minutes, taking a deep slow breath as you need. This technique, referred to as Brahmaree Pranayama, sets a vibration within the body that has immediate relaxing benefits. It will calm the mind, reset the nervous system, and induce melatonin.

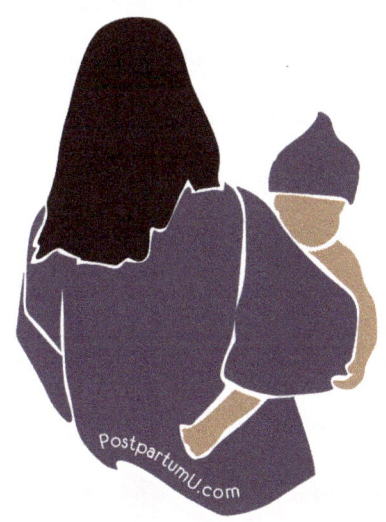

Magnesium Salt Bath

You may find comfort in taking a soak. Add some magnesium salt, herbs, or even some lavender oil. Just be careful not to fall asleep in the water!

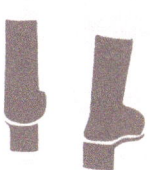

Healing, well-being, and living in your purpose begins with creating rhythm and ritual for it in your life.

Meditation

Meditation comes in many forms. From emptying your mind of thoughts (a skill to be practiced and learned) to focusing on your breathing or a specific mantra, there are many ways to fall into a more relaxed state of being. Use an app on your phone or practice in silence as you lay in bed.

Massage is an amazing technique for relaxation and sleep.

When to Seek Help

If you're unable to get to sleep because of constant recurring thoughts that feel scary, or recurring images or thoughts about a traumatic birth, it may be time to seek additional support from a professional such as a counselor, therapist, or other provider. If your baby is unable to sleep in stretches longer than two hours in a given day, consider chiropractic care to assess for possible causes.

4. Nervous System

You'll learn:

- The Root of Mental Health Concerns
- The Impact of Trauma
- Using Art to Heal
- Powerful Affirmations
- Postpartum Journaling

Chapter Four

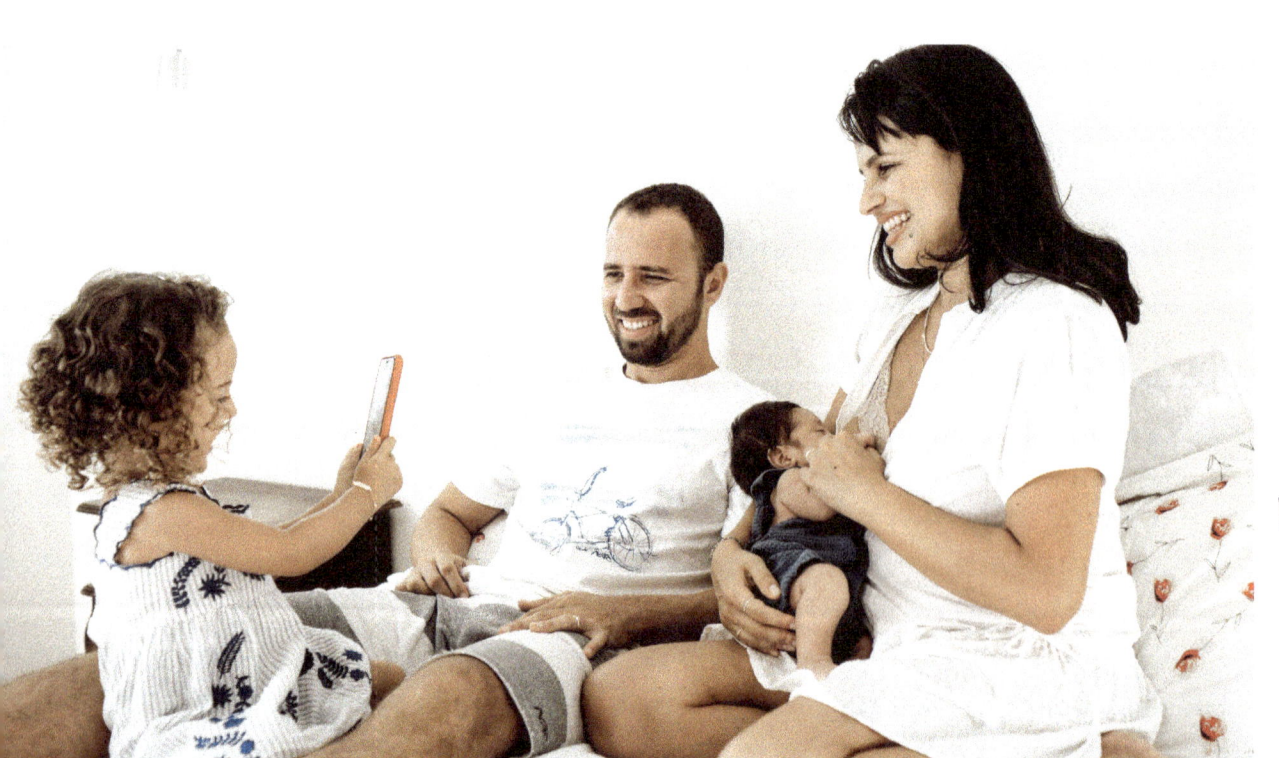

Nervous System: Postpartum

The nervous system is one of the most fascinating parts of the body, and one that is grossly overlooked in the postpartum years. The birth of a baby signals many changes to the body, including that of the nervous system. This special system is the communication powerhouse of your entire body, and its changes during and after birth shape the way you connect with your baby, digest your food, and even balance your hormones.

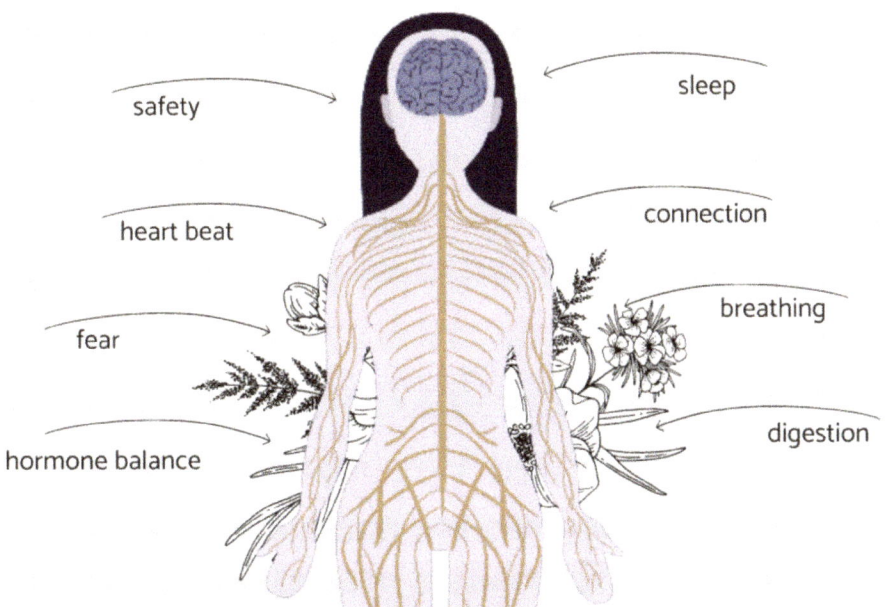

The millions of communication networks within your body are there to support your life and keep you safe. It's responsible for your automatic functions like your heart beating and breathing, and also responsible for your fight, flight, freeze, or fawn reactions when faced with danger. In postpartum, your biological norm is to have a nervous system that is on higher alert so that you can keep yourself and your baby safe from danger.

However, a sensitive nervous system can be troublesome when not supported or given the right signals of safety. Lack of nutrition, sleep, and support can also trigger a body into feeling unsafe and unsupported. When the nervous system is triggered to respond to what it feels is unsafe, it can send a cascade of emotions of upset, fear, frustration, anxiety, and even depression. A heightened nervous system can be responsible for irrational thoughts and fears, constant fatigue, poor digestion and stomach issues, trouble sleeping, hormone imbalance, and so much more.

To top it off, any sort of trauma can increase the sensitivity of your nervous system even more. Birth trauma accounts for over 45% of births in the United States alone. For many, the welcoming of their sweet child is blanketed in deep emotions and pain. Many postpartum women also feel a remembering of past traumas dating back to early childhood. Because the birth of a baby has the ability to open us to the most vulnerable parts of who we are, the work of healing becomes that much more important.

Not only are women faced with lack of support, proper nutrition, and sleep, life stress in today's world is at an all-time high. Societal pressures to get back to work, return to your pre-pregnancy weight quickly, misleading dieting fads that cause major depletion, and complete lack of emotional and physical support has many nervous systems on the brink of disaster. It's no wonder rates of depression and anxiety among mothers are rising exponentially.

Personal Story: Zaria M.

20 months into her first postpartum experience, Zaria M. didn't know where else to turn. Very quickly after the birth of her son, her hormones felt like they took a dive for the worst. She was experiencing high levels of anxiety, nausea, and diarrhea with ovulation, and even worse pains during the start of her period. Her fatigue and exhaustion were so high, that she felt the strain in her relationship and was unable to see clients as an Ayurvedic practitioner within her own practice.

As a vegan, eating the foods within the Postpartum Nutrition Plan wasn't something Zaria initially felt comfortable doing. However, in our next session together, she shared that she had decided to try chicken broth in secrecy and was amazing at how soothed she felt. Although I always recommend taking things slow with such a major dietary change, she was well in tune with the body and continued to add in animal foods as she felt comfortable.

With more sessions, Zaria continued uncovering major insights to her new life and her identity as a woman, mother, partner, and practitioner. Using what's outlined in this book, she uncovered her fears of getting pregnant again that ultimately contributed to her ovulation sickness (by keeping her partner away because she was ill, she could help prevent pregnancy).

Of course, in a matter of a few short months, Zaria changed her entire life around. All symptoms surrounding her menstrual cycle had disappeared. Her color, vibrancy, and energy had returned, and her relationship with her partner and son felt full for the first time since pregnancy. She also made a fresh start in her practice with a new vision of health and immediately saw her efforts with her own clients as successful in just a short period of time.

Personal Story: Amy T.

Amy had been suffering for 5 long years after the birth of her baby. She struggled with losing weight, constant fatigue and exhaustion, diarrhea, migraines, and around the 2 year mark, she was diagnosed with a "mild fatty liver." From there, the vaginal yeast infections came full force. Nearly every month for 3 solid years, Amy struggled with yeast. She saw a number of doctors, took all the medications possible, took numerous tests with nothing to report, and felt "hopeless and helpless."

Amy hired me as a last-ditch effort. Immediately, we found nutrient-dense favorable meals that fit into her Indian cultural food practices. We added healing spiced teas to her daily regimen as well, and explored many emotions and feelings that had been stored way inside her for years.

Although her emotional health seemed to improve, Amy's infections continued on. With a bit of focus, we honed in and discovered that she was highly allergic to garlic, which she was using to combat the yeast. After removing the garlic from her life, her infections ceased. It took a few more weeks of healing, nourishing, and detoxing for overall whole-body improvements.

By 4 months in, Amy had made a nearly full recovery. She no longer had migraines, diarrhea, or constant battles with fatigue and exhaustion. She was losing weight and her periods were easier as well. In an interview with Amy, she shared with me for the first time that her symptoms had originally been so bad, that she planned to end her life if she didn't get better after our sessions together. From her experience, she discovered her love and passion for nourishment. She later enrolled in a nutrition program for her new career change so that she could begin helping women heal their bodies after baby.

You can hear Amy's story in her own words (along with many others) on the Postpartum University® Podcast Episode 11.

Personal Story: Megan B.

Megan came to me for the sole purpose of supporting her with food to heal her gut. Since around 3 months postpartum, her tummy had been reacting to certain foods. She wasn't able to pinpoint what foods were triggering for her, but the bloating, gas, digestive upset, and exhaustion felt terrible. The Postpartum Recovery Assessment gave her a score of "moderate" imbalance. Her lab work showed nothing abnormal and she was desperate for support.

First, Megan eliminated both gluten and diary from her

diet and began eating the recipes from the Postpartum Nutrition Plan. Although her bloating and digestive upset felt a bit better, her energy reduced and she was nervous that something wasn't right. With a bit of reassurance and encouragement to allow her body rest, Megan began feeling better and better. By the end of the first week, her energy not only returned but also surpassed her expectations. She felt alert, clear-minded, and didn't need a mid-day nap.

Even more, Megan noticed something she didn't expect. Her daughter had constantly triggered her into angry screaming that felt out of control. But since starting the Postpartum Nutrition Plan, she had not felt rage or anger or out of control! Her physical symptoms no longer existed, her energy returned, and she felt more connected and in touch with her own needs and the needs of her children and family.

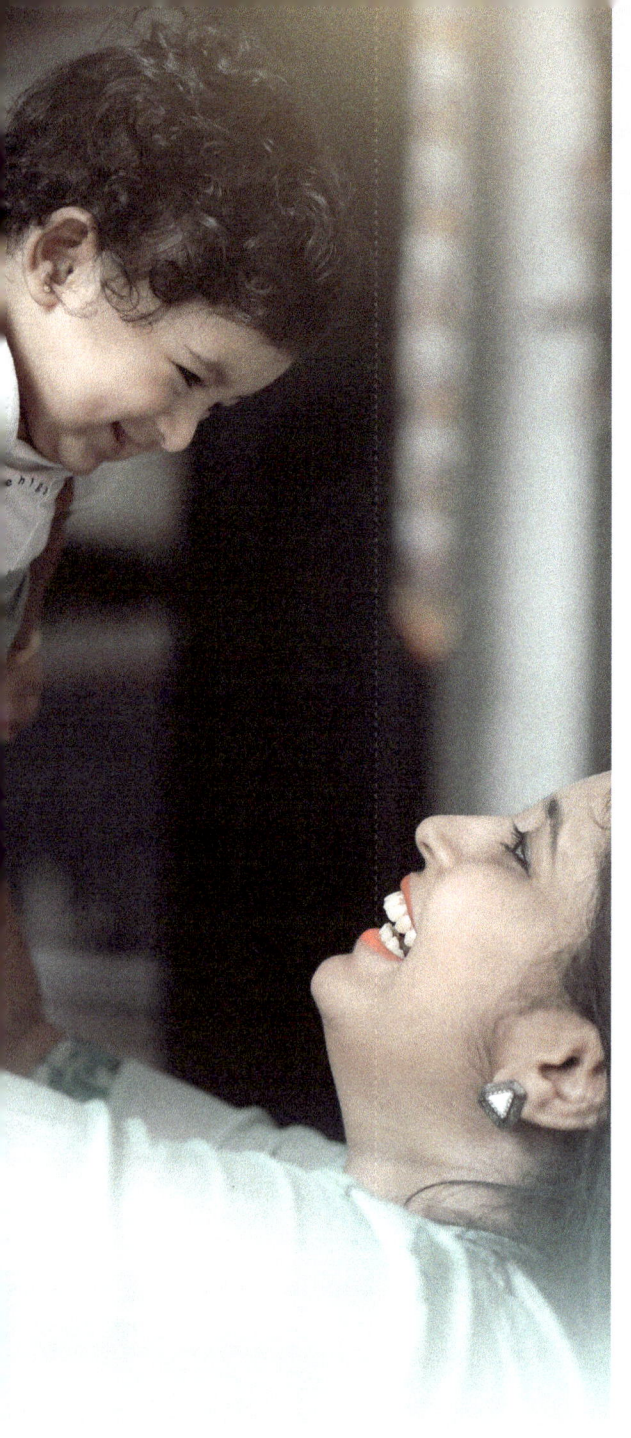

Releasing Stored Trauma

As a biological protective mechanism to keep you safe, your body stores trauma within the cells of your body. Every time you hear, see, smell, remember, or even feel something that reminds your cells of trauma or extreme stress, it can trigger your body into a state of reactivity (fight, flight, freeze, or fawn). A flow of emotions and feelings related to the trauma can occur in a matter of seconds, leaving you feeling completely out of control.

There are many ways to heal from trauma. Working with a professional, journaling, and participating in art therapy are just some of the ways my clients have worked through their trauma. I have listed some of my favorite methods of releasing trauma and regulating your nervous system within this chapter of the book. Explore what feels best for you and be sure to look for other avenues of healing if you need, including EMDR and somatic therapy.

One of the most effective ways to release stored trauma within the body is through a technique called Tension and Trauma Releasing Exercise Therapy (TRE ® Therapy). This is an exercise that you can do in the comfort of your own home and is often referred to as Shake Therapy. Although not highly researched, its wide range of benefits cannot go unnoticed, and it poses zero risk to anyone who does it.

This therapy uses the body's natural tension release processes to help the body reduce the stored trauma within, and supports the nervous system in recalibrating to a healthier, less reactive base point. You can learn more about how to do this exercise on our website (www.PostpartumU.com/Workbook) or via internet videos or a trained provider.

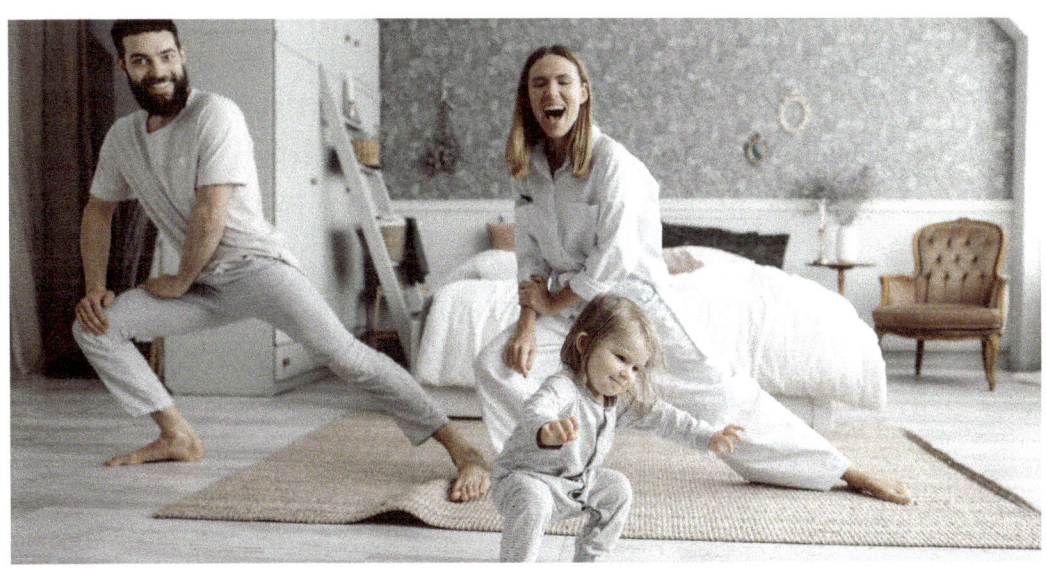

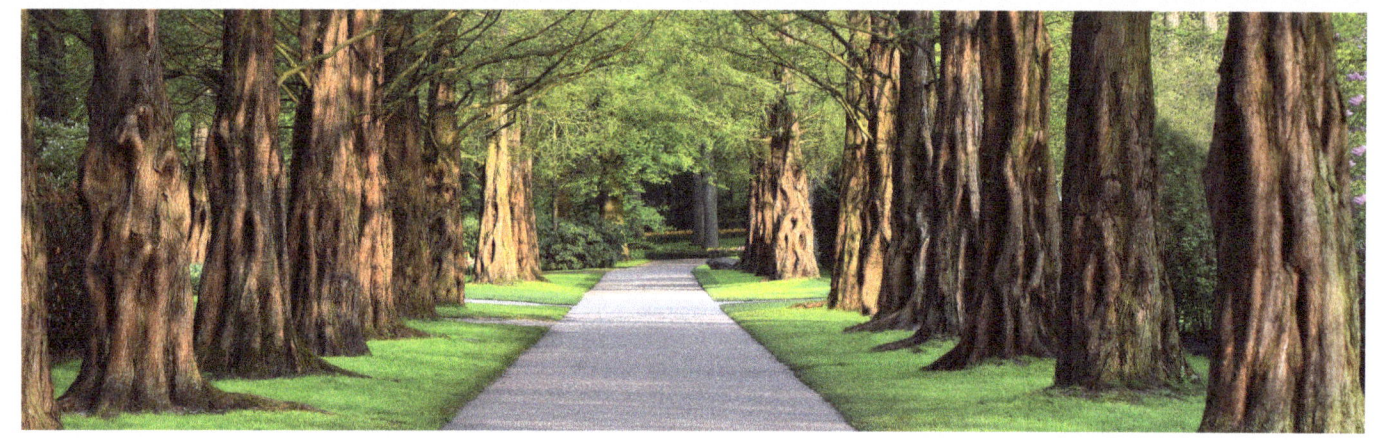

Nature is therapy.

Sitting in the green grass is grounding. Taking a walk in the woods is mind clearing. Nature has this funny way of resetting our body and bringing us back into ourselves.

On a spiritual level, you could say that as mothers, we need to connect with the roots of our being, connecting with Mother Nature, mother-to-mother. You could also say that being in nature brings life back into us; a place where we are nourished at the most fundamental level.

Whatever the reason is, we know, without a shadow of a doubt, that being with nature (in any form) lowers your blood pressure, decreases stress hormones, and stimulates the immune system (even to the point of expressing anti-cancer proteins). Sometimes, we just need a gentle reminder to bring you back into what matters most.

"It must be hormones..."

Major hair loss, mood swings, menstrual pain, constant headaches, fatigue, depression, anxiety, weight gain…the list of symptoms of hormone imbalance often seems unending. And they are the first to blame anytime you don't feel well. "It must be hormones" is a consistent statement we hear from our partners, medical providers, mothers, and even ourselves.

It's true that hormones play a significant part in the functionality of your body, especially in relation to pregnancy, birth, and postpartum. As explained in the other sections of this guide, a postpartum body has very specific needs to address that are far different than any other period in a woman's life.

It's also important to note that the immune system is regulated by your hormones, and your nervous system plays a special role in supporting your hormones. So if you are experiencing imbalances, you can bet that other functions within you are also experiencing imbalances.

Postpartum hormones are not naturally out of balance. After the birth of your baby, hormones are in a natural state of fluctuation. They are doing what is biologically necessary to support you and your infant.

The imbalance of hormones occurs when this natural shift isn't properly supported (an art that has been lost through the generations). When you don't get the nutrients and sleep you need (and the knowledge and support to make it happen), your hormones begin to feel unstable. If there is trauma or stress involved, those hormones may feel completely out of control before you've even had a chance to blink.

Often, by getting the rest and the nutrition you need, your hormones tend to level out and feel more at peace. However, there are times when no amount of sleep or well absorbed nutrients will help.

For this, I highly recommend addressing imbalances from the very root. Using therapies such as medications, essential oils, CBD oil, and so on are tools that can help, but they are simply coping strategies and don't address the actual root problem or promote lasting healing. To do this, it's essential to begin healing the nervous system.

> Postpartum hormones are not naturally out of balance.

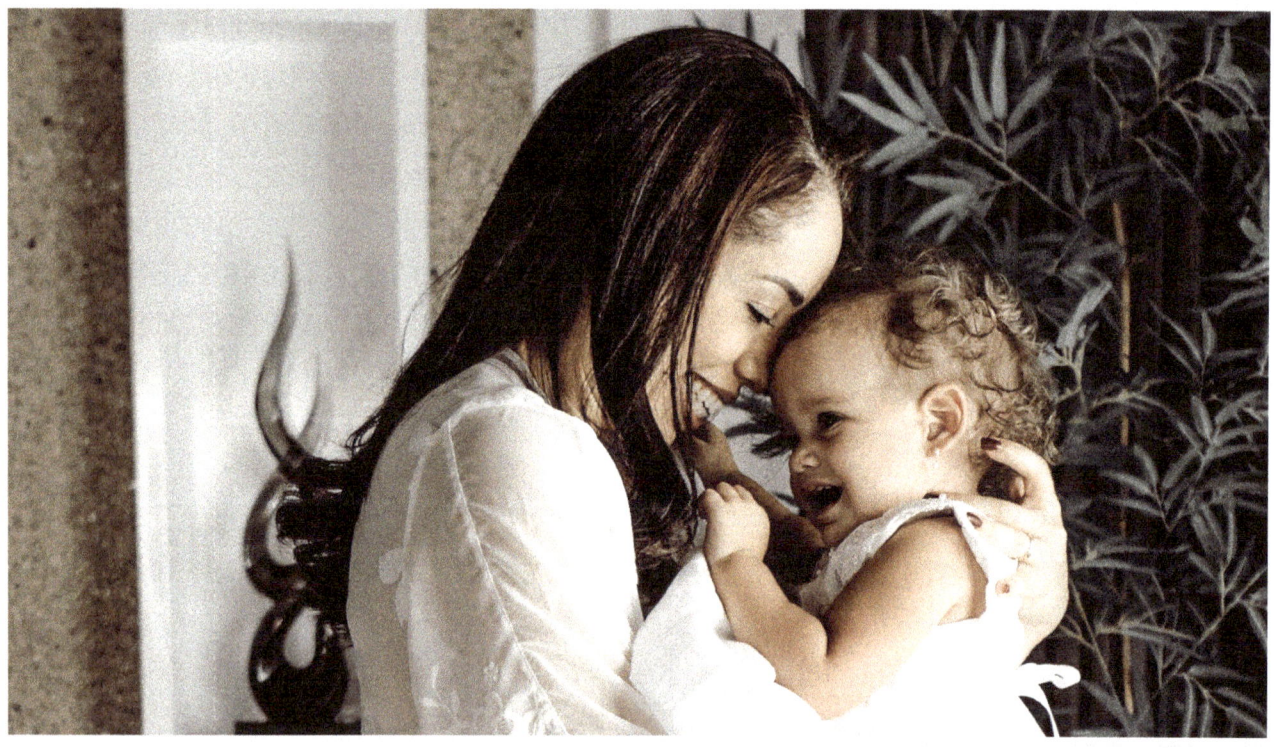

4 Reasons for Lingering Hormone Imbalance After Food, Rest, and Emotional Support Are Met:

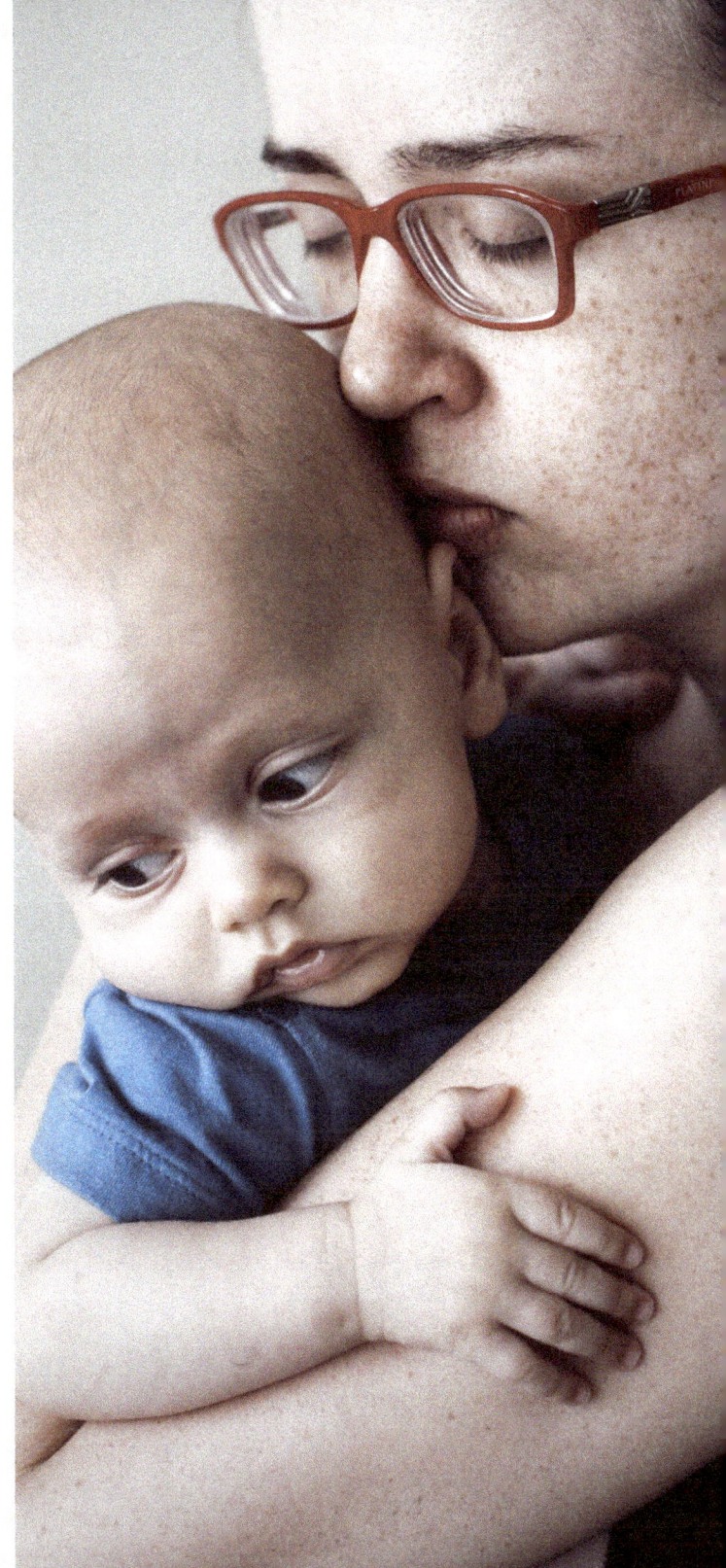

1. Trauma

Trauma, whether from pregnancy or birth or life before baby, can have a lasting impact on hormone balance. It's important to be actively resolving and healing from any life trauma that has come to you, no matter how small you think it is. Trauma and any difficult situation that have left long negative imprints within you change your brain chemistry and even how your body functions. Actively seek avenues for healing.

2. Negative Self-Talk

When there is constant negativity, it's easy to get thrown into a negative spiral that may feel like depression (or even make depression worse). Listen to the thoughts that are coming to you. If you are always telling yourself that you are "no good" or "stupid" or "ugly," you will only create more of that in your life to prove you're correct (this is just how psychology works). Negative self-talk is a terrible cycle that many don't notice they're in until it's become a deeply ingrained habit. Speak kindly to yourself and use affirmations to help you. Journal often on it as things come up to help release the negative beliefs.

3. Unexpressed/Suppressed Feelings

Women have been told throughout history that emotions are "bad" and that feelings are simply "hormonal." Because of this, women tend to hold back, force down their feelings, and remain quiet. This leads to big emotions like anger, rage, resentment, panic attacks, and more. These are surface emotions that feel out of control and are usually hiding deeper, more painful feelings (such as sadness, despair, feelings of unworthiness, and so on). Allow yourself to feel big emotions and get them out of your body. Holding onto emotions can increase powerlessness and negatively impact your body's healing journey.

4. Underlying Thyroid Problems

Nearly 1 out of every 7 women experiences thyroid problems postpartum. There is a direct correlation between autoimmune issues of the thyroid and postpartum depression and/or anxiety. However, when an autoimmune issue arises during life after childbirth, it's a sign that the body has been in a state of ill health for some time. Actively use this guide to support your health and consider support from a medical professional. It's important to ask the question: *WHY is the thyroid out of balance in postpartum for so many?* The answer is not because you had a baby. Its root is in the fact that you have had little care and support in the way in which your body needed it most. To reverse that, you must go back and give your body what it needs most: nourishment, sleep, and emotional support.

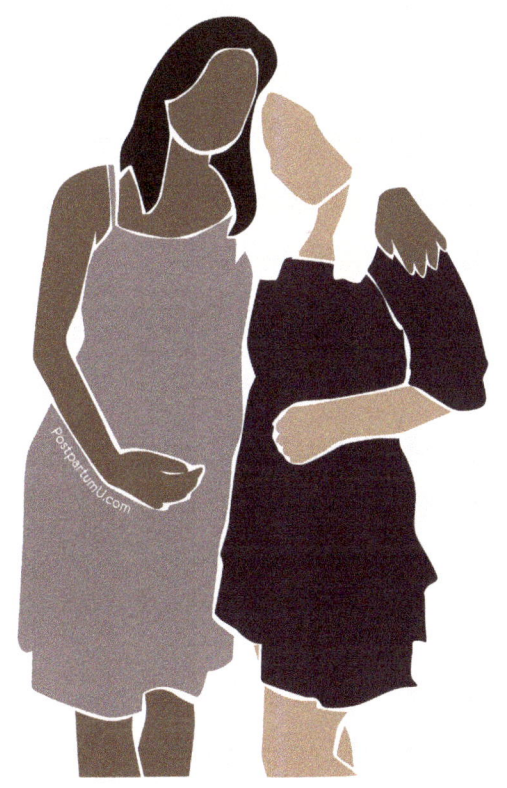

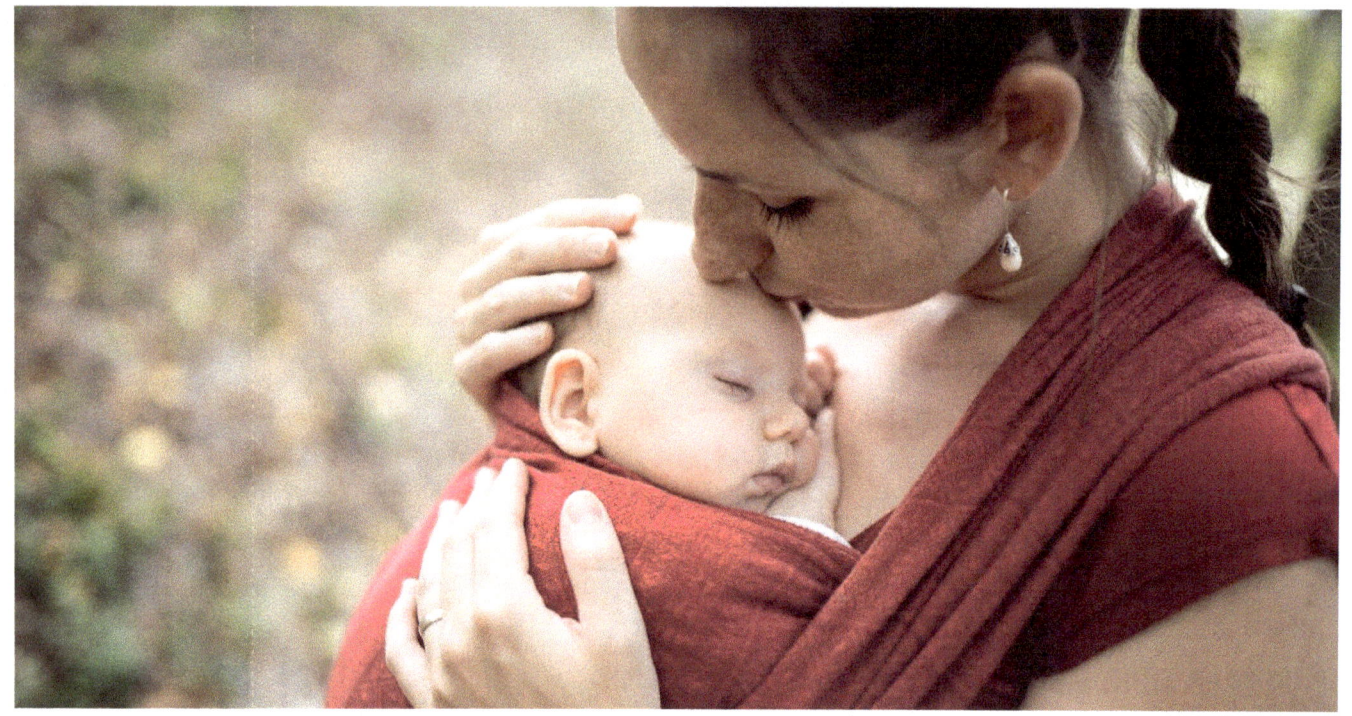

For many women, the path to hormone imbalance is slow and steady. Most women realize they are in need of additional support right around the time toddlerhood comes. This is because your babe gets a bit more independent and you find yourself with some breathing room. This is the very reason why most of my clients are 2-3 years postpartum.

It's also the time that addressing hormonal imbalance becomes incredibly urgent, because, after about 4 years, the symptoms you are experiencing notoriously transform into something far more complicated. This is the time when your body decides that this may be your new state of normal, and it will carry you through menopause.

It isn't that you are a new person in postpartum, it's that you are closer to the person you are within your heart.

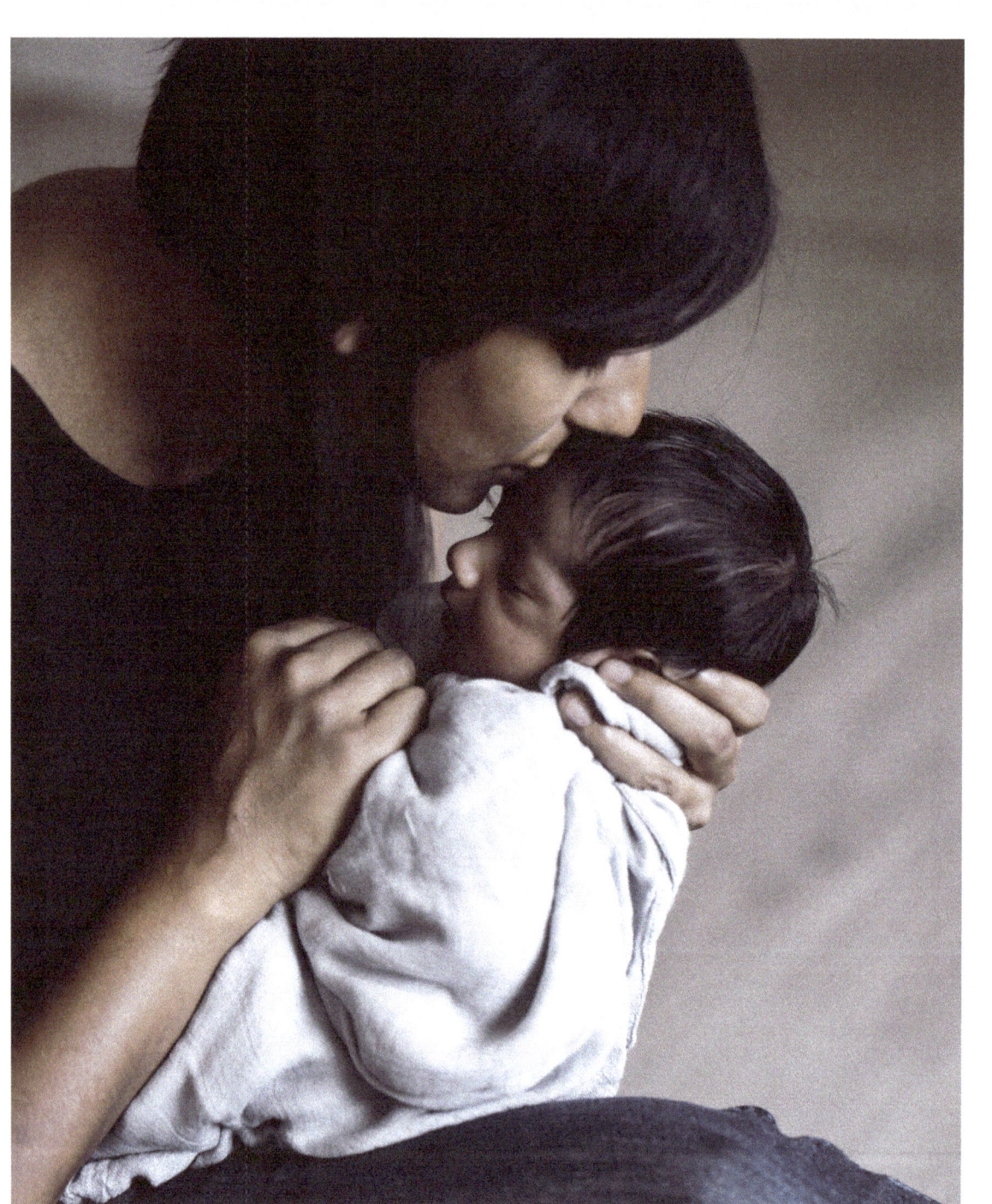

Nervous System Healing + the Arts

Using Art for Emotion and Trauma Healing

In working through my own trauma and emotional battles, as well as working with hundreds of women through theirs, I have found a direct correlation between many of the physical symptoms of hormone imbalance, dis-ease, and more and the emotional state of the body.

Lousie Hay, an author, healer, and minister, relates most of the symptoms and dis-eases in her book *You Can Heal Your Life* to the experiences, thoughts, and emotions that we experience. You can find a list of symptoms as they relate to emotion in her book. For example, she states that migraines relate to a dislike of being driven, or period pain is the rejection of one's femininity with guilt and fear.

Although her reasoning behind the symptoms may not always make sense for you (although they nearly always do for me and my clients), they teach us how interconnected our mind and body are.

Remember that emotions are tools that guide you through what's going on within you. They are NOT who you are, but a simple representation of your needs.

Using art is an amazing tool to dive into the subconscious.

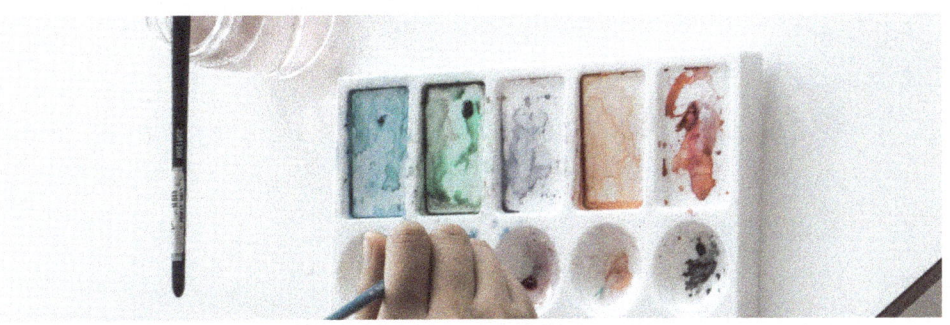

One way to approach understanding on a deeper level is using art for your healing. Art Therapy has been around for a long time. I am trained specifically in birth and postpartum related art healing. During my training, the main lesson was that you have the ability to heal your body already within you. Just as you heal a physical wound, you can heal emotional wounds as well.

Using art is an amazing tool to dive into the subconscious and understand more about what lies beneath. You can access the thoughts and feelings that you haven't been able to put to words or that you didn't know were influencing your thoughts and decisions.

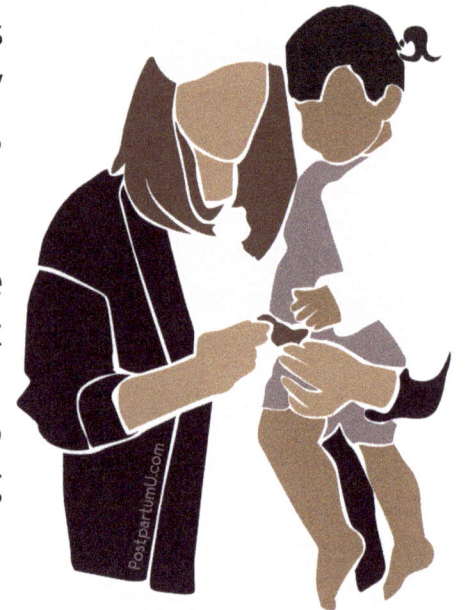

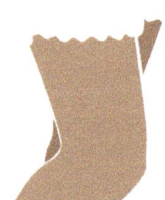

To use art to dive deeper into your emotions, I highly recommend paint, watercolor, or pastels. Get out all your materials and a large paper. Don't have any preconceived ideas about what you want to create. Instead, sit with your paper for a second and think up an open-ended question. The more random it feels, the better, because you will not have formed an idea around what you will create with your art. Instead, your art will develop and flow naturally.

As you paint or draw your response to your question, you'll come across a time when you feel you can't make anything else. Don't stop. This is the point where you will be able to reach into your subconscious. Whatever you do, keep your brush or pastel to paper and move it. When you feel done from that, step back and journal your experience. You'll be surprised at what you learn.

Some example questions you can form your art with:
- What does is mean to be a mother?
- Draw the landscape of your heart.
- Describe the feeling of safety with your art.

This may be an exercise that is best done with a trained person who can help facilitate your healing. Try it, and if you don't feel you've experienced a major breakthrough, find a local person trained in art therapy to support you. You can also go to www.PostpartumU.com/Workbook for more information.

Back to the Roots

A Story from Around the World

In **China**, *zuo yuezi* represents a full month-long restorative period for new mothers. Zuo yuezi means "sitting of the month," a period in which a mother moves from life before baby to life with baby. During this healing time, only soups, stews, and broths are consumed to support overall healing, hormone balance, and a healthy milk supply. No cold drinks or raw foods are allowed. Female family members come to the home to cook meals, take care of household tasks, and make sure the mother is sleeping well. This will support the re-balancing of chi energy that had been lost during birth and help her get stronger so she can return to her family healthy and well.

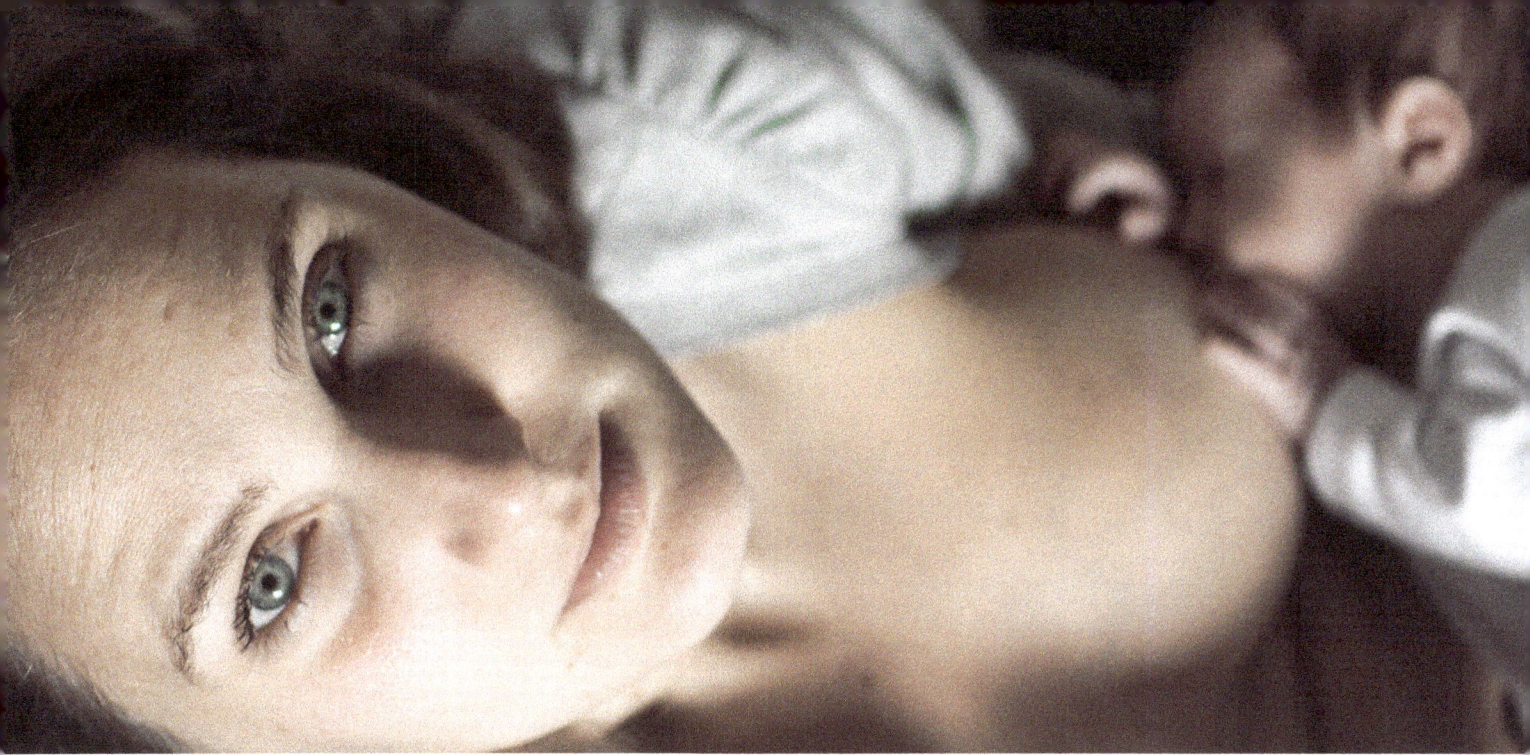

Affirmations for Motherhood

Affirmations are powerful tools that can support you as a mother by changing the way you think and feel. Many ups and downs of hormones are controlled by the thoughts you think and the feelings you have. Affirmations are ways to "reprogram" your brain and train yourself to feel better. Although they are not a cure-all, they are an amazing tool to add as you shift and change into the mother you wish to become.

To use these affirmations, you can write them out on sticky notes and set them around the house, being sure to say them out loud every time you see them. Or you can simply pick your top 3 and make a point to write them and repeat them out loud several times a day.

Affirmations

I recognize my feelings and thoughts as tools that guide me to lead a better life.

I am the best mom for my baby.

My intuition guides me to the right choices every time.

I embrace today with open arms. I can do this.

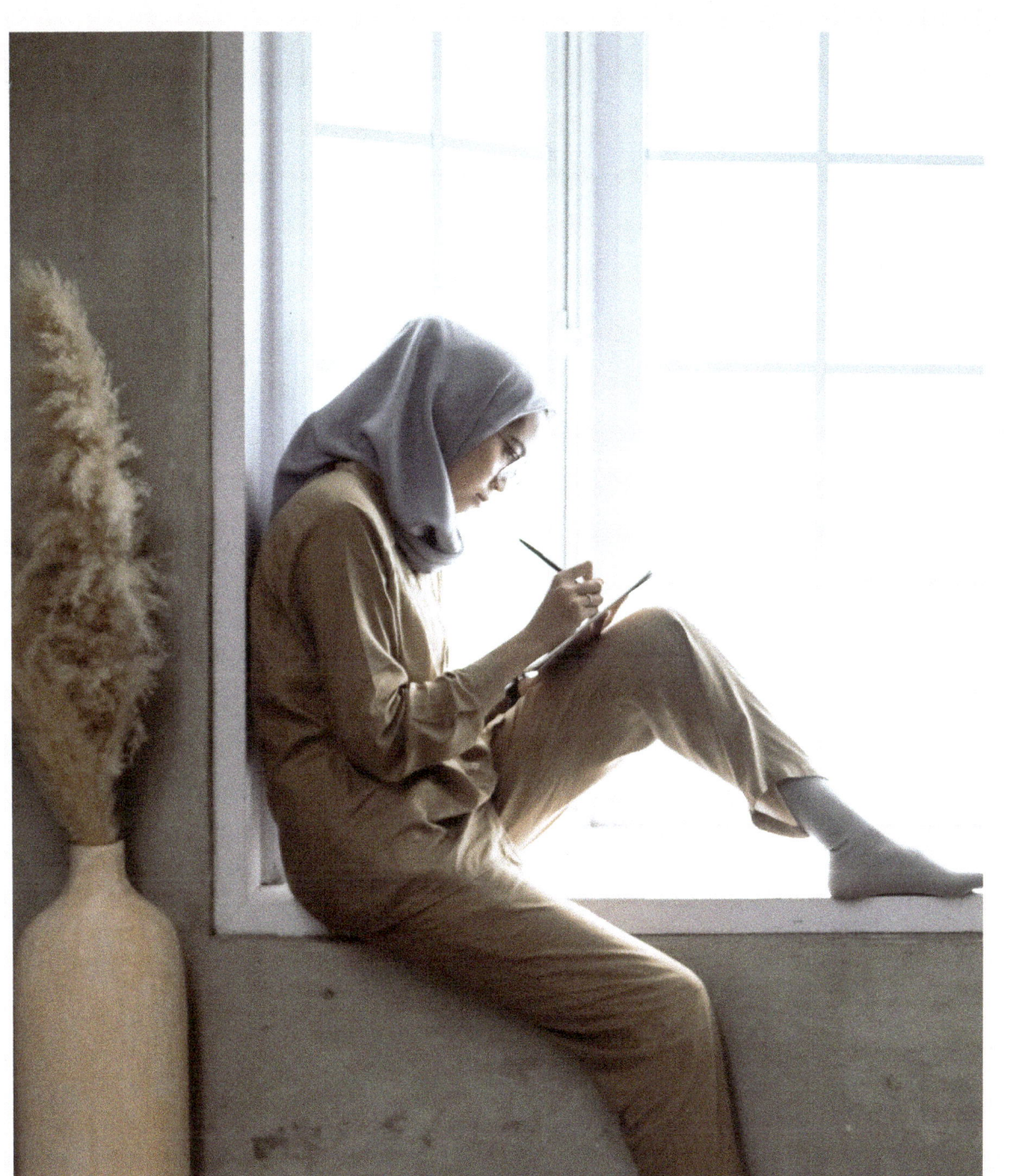

The Power of Journaling

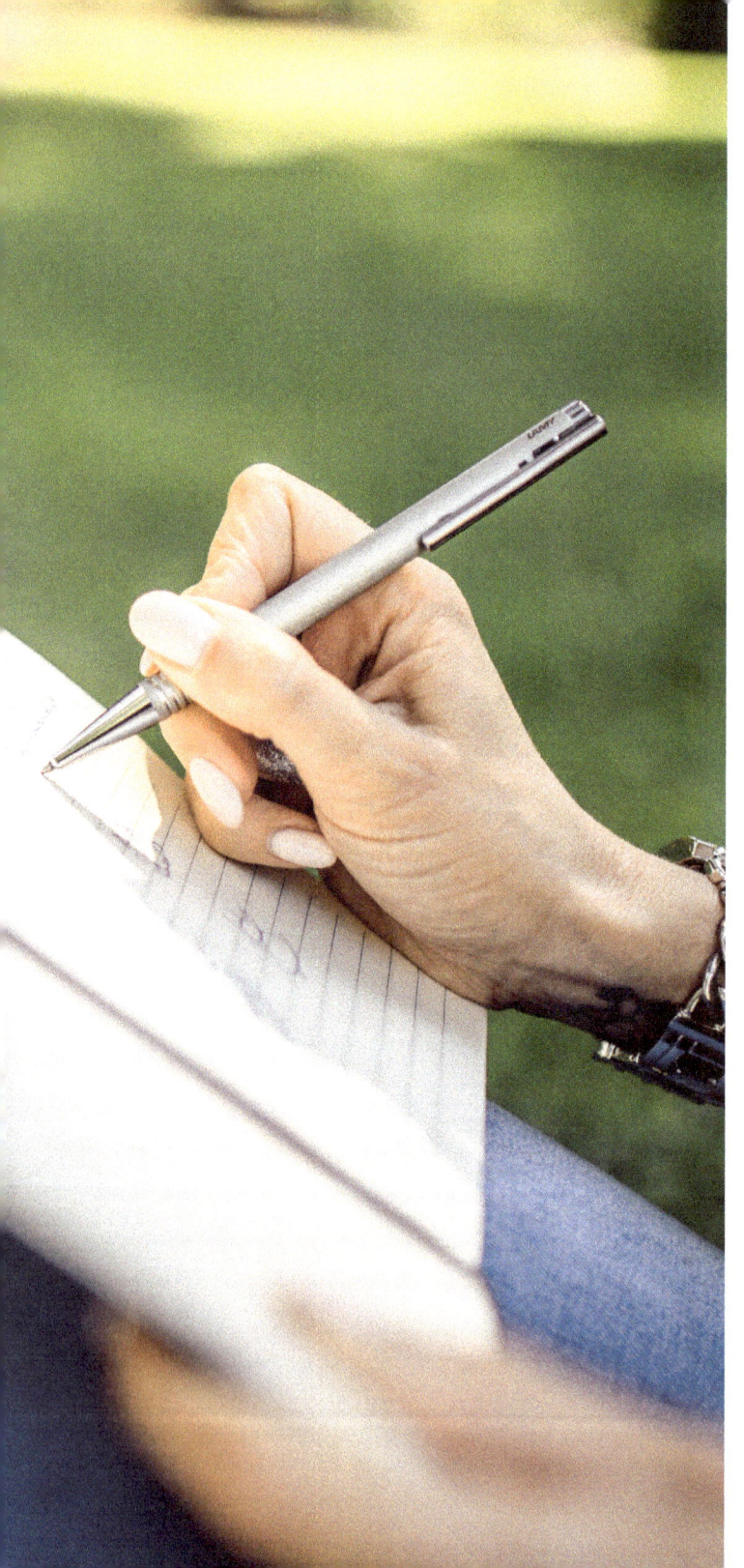

Journaling to Heal

Journaling is the key to all things that reside within you. After you give birth, all the things you once knew completely shift and change. Who you are becomes radically different, and the first several years after birth are about discovering who that person is.

These questions are potent tools supporting you in your transformation into a better person. Grab a journal specific to your postpartum exploration and simply write, without worry of it being read, seen, or what kind of "mistakes" you make. Simply write everything that comes through your pen from your heart, and then watch as you release and see the person you are becoming. It's absolutely eye-opening.

What's one thing you can do for yourself today that will bring you joy?

_____

_____

_____

_____

_____

_____

_____

_____

_____

_____

_____

How can you express more love for your body?

_____
_____
_____
_____
_____
_____
_____
_____
_____
_____
_____

What do you feel is your biggest strength as a mother?

Download 30+ journal prompts here:

www.PostpartumU.com/Workbook

5. Rhythms

You'll learn:
- Rhythms and Cycles
- Moon Connection
- Tracking Your Cycles

Chapter Five

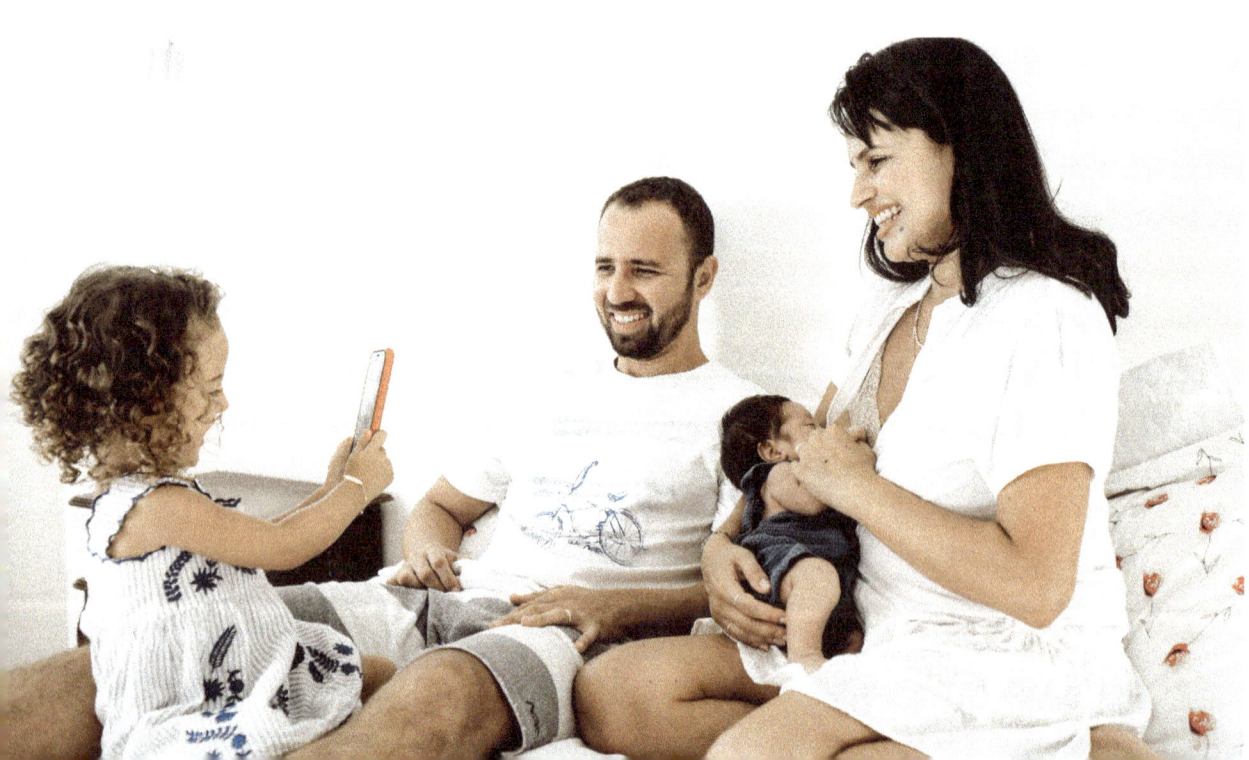

Following the Rhythms and Cycles of Life and Motherhood

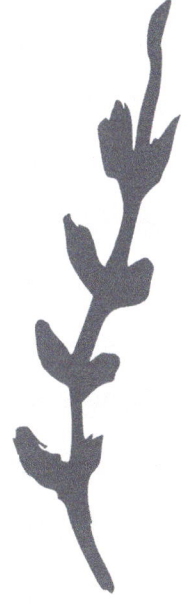

Everything in life follows a cyclical rhythm - the seasons, tides, moon, ecosystems, life/death. Even our heartbeat, menstruation, the life of cells, and everything in between follows a rhythm and cycle. As mothers, we are a part of this ever-moving rhythm. The more we accept, honor, and flow with it, the easier the journey.

Nature offers us a profound connection to the natural ebb and flow of life and supports a deeper connection to our own biological rhythms. Chronobiology is a field that studies our body's natural biological cycles, including mental, physical, emotional, circadian, hormonal, and menstruation, especially in relationship to nature and the solar and lunar cycles. In short, the human body is greatly influenced by the rhythms and cycles of the world, and in motherhood, we are even more sensitive to such intricate dances of life.

When we connect to these natural rhythms, we can begin to not only deepen our understanding of them, but also support these beautiful parts of who we are and honor them. You can use these to help you understand your body, advocate for your needs, and give yourself permission to let go, step back, say yes or no, and simply be more in the moment with who you are (so that you can be with your children more in the process).

Women and the Moon

Menstruation is derived from the Latin and Greek word for moon. In ancient Greece, it was believed that during the time of menstruation, women were spiritually and mentally more powerful. What we actually see throughout history are stories from cultures around the world that say the exact same thing. We even have entire rituals and traditions that have been derived from knowing that the moon impacts fertility, as well as our emotions, our behavior, and our sleep.

This cyclical nature that our body follows is an instrumental tool to finding our own health and well-being. Specifically, our world does not honor the rhythm of the female body, which is vastly different than the male. The masculine approach to constantly be on the go does not fit in to the female body and its need for rest, activity, creative expression, and reflection.

It's no wonder women consistently burn out, get sick, and feel completely overwhelmed. We're not living in our cycle. In order to fully understand your own body, in order to find your own ebb and flow, you must understand its natural rhythms and honor them.

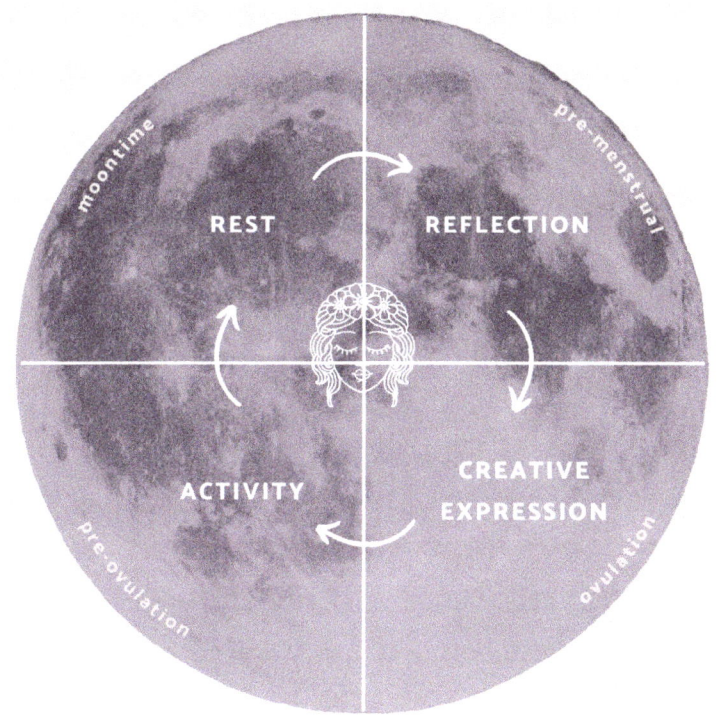

Your own cycle may not necessarily line up with the moon itself, but tracking will help you understand better where you are and what you need. You may find that it all lines up for you as you get your body back into health and balance, but know that that is not necessary. Track your physical and emotional symptoms within each month and get to know your unique rhythms, even if you are shifting and changing, as we do in postpartum.

The goal is to have a life where you love and honor your body and its needs. A life where you can very easily say, "*I remember when that happens, then I'm going to have to make this kind of shift in order to be back on track, to be back in the rhythm of my own body*". It is a beautiful gift.

Tracking Rhythms

Part of self-love is following the rhythms of your body so that you become intimately knowledgeable in all things YOU.

Your menstrual cycle, your hormones, your cravings, your energy, and more are all in a cycle with the moon and within the seasons. Find a cycle journal, or use the one in this book, to take note of the rhythms of your body and honor what comes up.

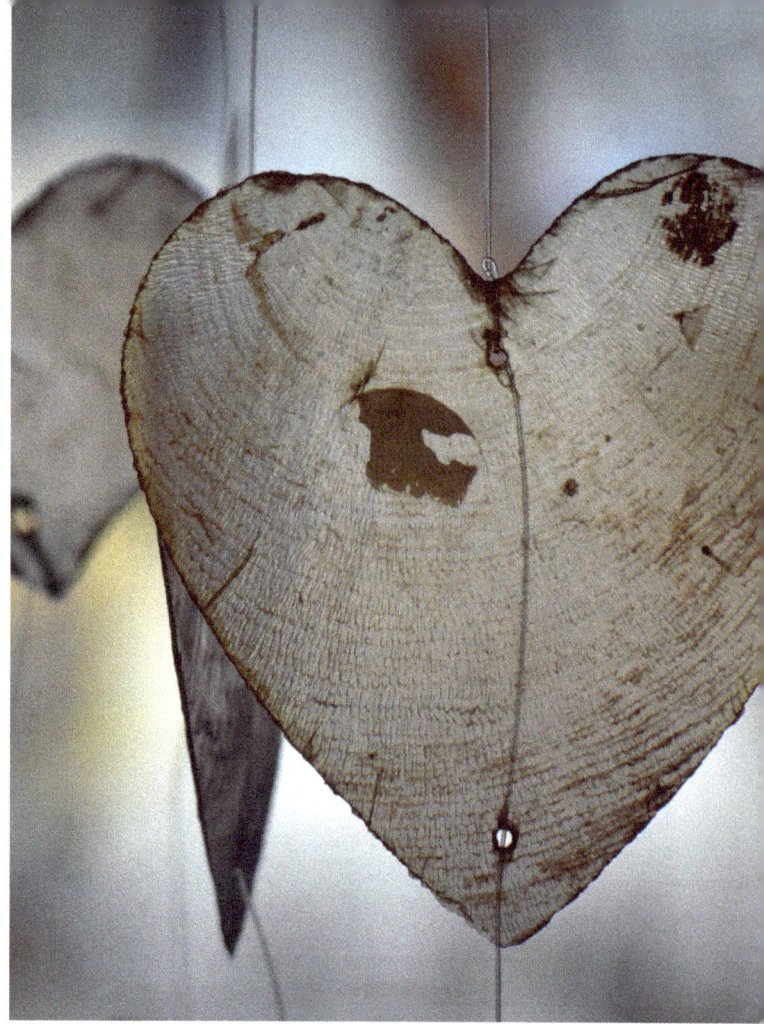

Learning to love yourself at such a deep level - to truly accept yourself - is known as some of the hardest work on the planet.

It's an ongoing relationship and never-ending pursuit of self-love.

Shade in, use colors or symbols, and simply have fun tracking (there is no right/wrong way)!

Day	1	2	3	4	5	6	7	8	9	10	11	12	13	14	15	16	17	18	19	20	21	22	23	24	25	26	27	28	29	30	31
Bleeding																															
Discharge																															
Acne																															
Bloating																															
Cramping																															
Breast Soreness																															
Achey																															
Diarrhea																															
Nausea/ Vomiting																															
Aroused																															
Happy/ Joyful																															
Sad/ Depressed																															
Fear / Anxiety																															
Foggy / Slow																															
Angry / Irritable																															
Calm / Content																															

Download this worksheet here:

Remember: Rituals and rhythms are a necessary part of life in motherhood.

Without them, feelings of disconnect and confusion set in, leaving you depleted and overwhelmed.

Powerful. Nurturing. Sacred. Complete.

Use this information to incorporate rituals and rhythms of healing and health in your family. Start by trying out many of the techniques listed in this guide and intertwine them into your daily life. Ask your family and children to join you when appropriate.

By making your health a priority, you show your family that YOU, as well as self-care, are important life skills. Self-care will naturally become community care.

Remember, the home center is you. You are the creator and hold the womb-space of your family. Therefore, everything you do will radiate outwardly to your partner, children, and beyond.

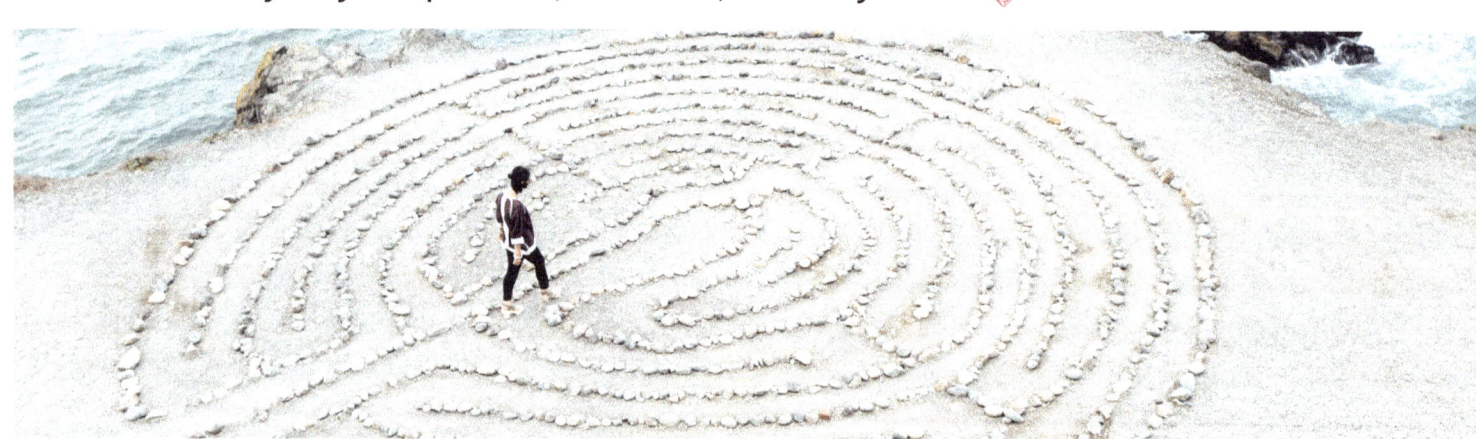

Movement

You'll learn:

- Movement to Heal
- Best Practices and Safety Guidelines
- Specific Exercises
- Cardio and Weightlifting

Bonus Chapter

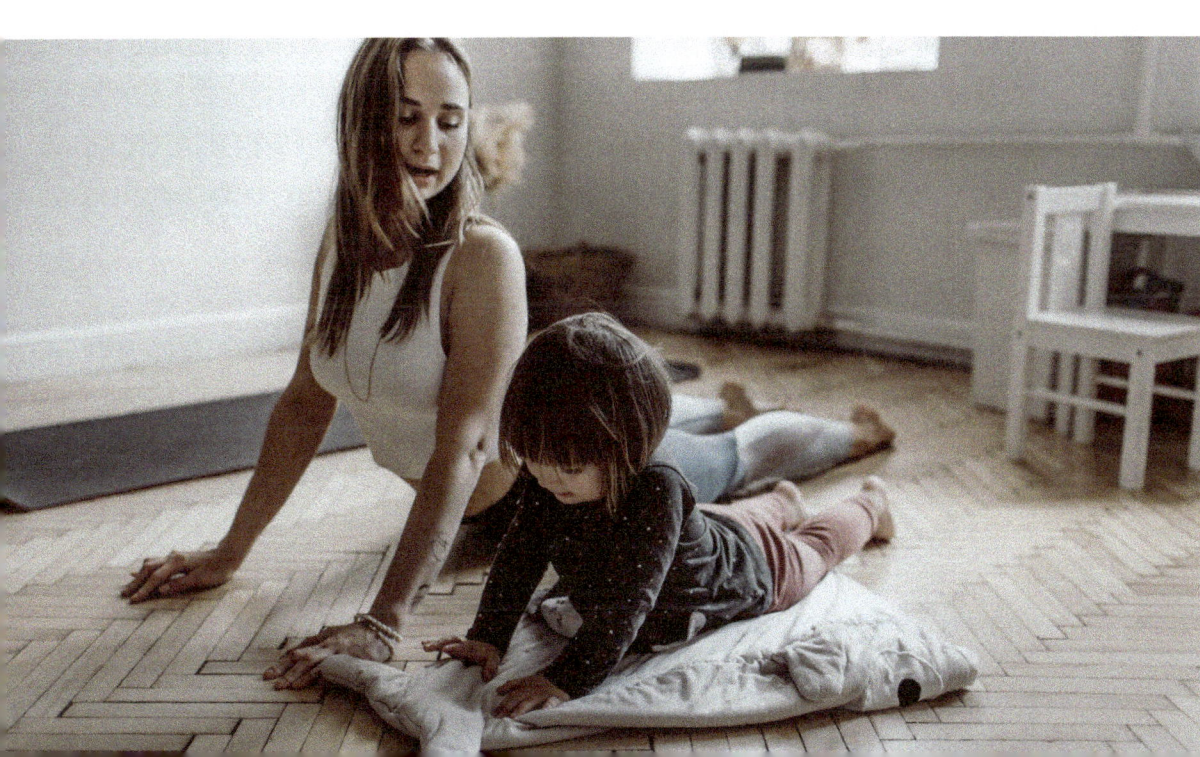

Postpartum exercise is one of the most heavily misguided areas of motherhood.

Shouts from the rooftops to "get your body back" and societal pressure to fit back into those pre-pregnancy jeans have a lot of women working out and feeling worse for it.

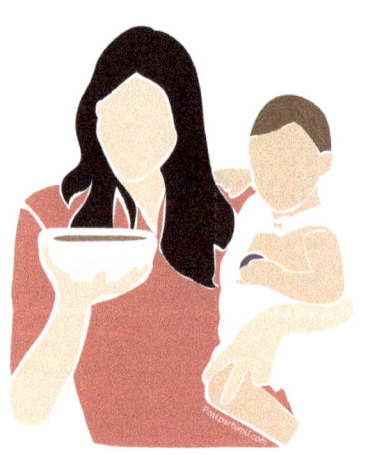

For most women, exercise after childbirth should be slow and gradual, even if exercise was part of your lifestyle before children. The physiological changes from pregnancy and birth leave your joints, organs, and ligaments in different places, stretched and vulnerable to injury. Even your pelvic bones remain in the birthing position for weeks, and if trauma was involved, years after childbirth.

Often, organ prolapse, diastasis recti (a splitting of the abdominal muscles), and urinary incontinence become issues because improper exercise practices are likely, and often exercise for postpartum begins too soon.

However, science and experience is clear: proper and safe exercising, even in the months and years after having a baby, provides a mother with a healthier immune system, better mood, and a major energy boost.

If you have organ prolapse (or suspect one), diastasis recti, or urinary incontinence, please see your local Pelvic Floor Physical Therapist who specializes in women's health, and do so before beginning a workout routine. They will be able to give you therapeutic exercises to resolve your specific issues and concerns.

If you are new to exercise, have a history of working out but are in the first 3 months postpartum, or you experience any of the symptoms mentioned above (or have had a cesarean), you can begin exercise by focusing on these areas (in order and shared in more detail in the next sections):

- Deep abdominal breathing
- Posture awareness
- Gentle stretching
- Closing yoga

Motherhood is learned. So is healing.

Keep in mind that much of what you do in your daily life already constitutes as exercise. Carrying a baby around all day, bouncing, swaying, carrying big car seats, shopping bags, and baby bags, chasing toddlers…much of this lifting, bending, and moving is already a workout! Be sure to cut yourself some slack. You are already doing the hard work of exercising.

Use the strategies I share with you here to make your daily moving more powerful in building strength, releasing toxins, promoting calm, and preventing physical damage.

Exercise is a tool for being the healthiest version of you. It's not about dropping all the weight or about returning back to your pre-pregnancy state. As a matter of fact, your body will never be the same after birth. Give yourself time to mourn this if you need to. Then move on to living within the best version of your body ever.

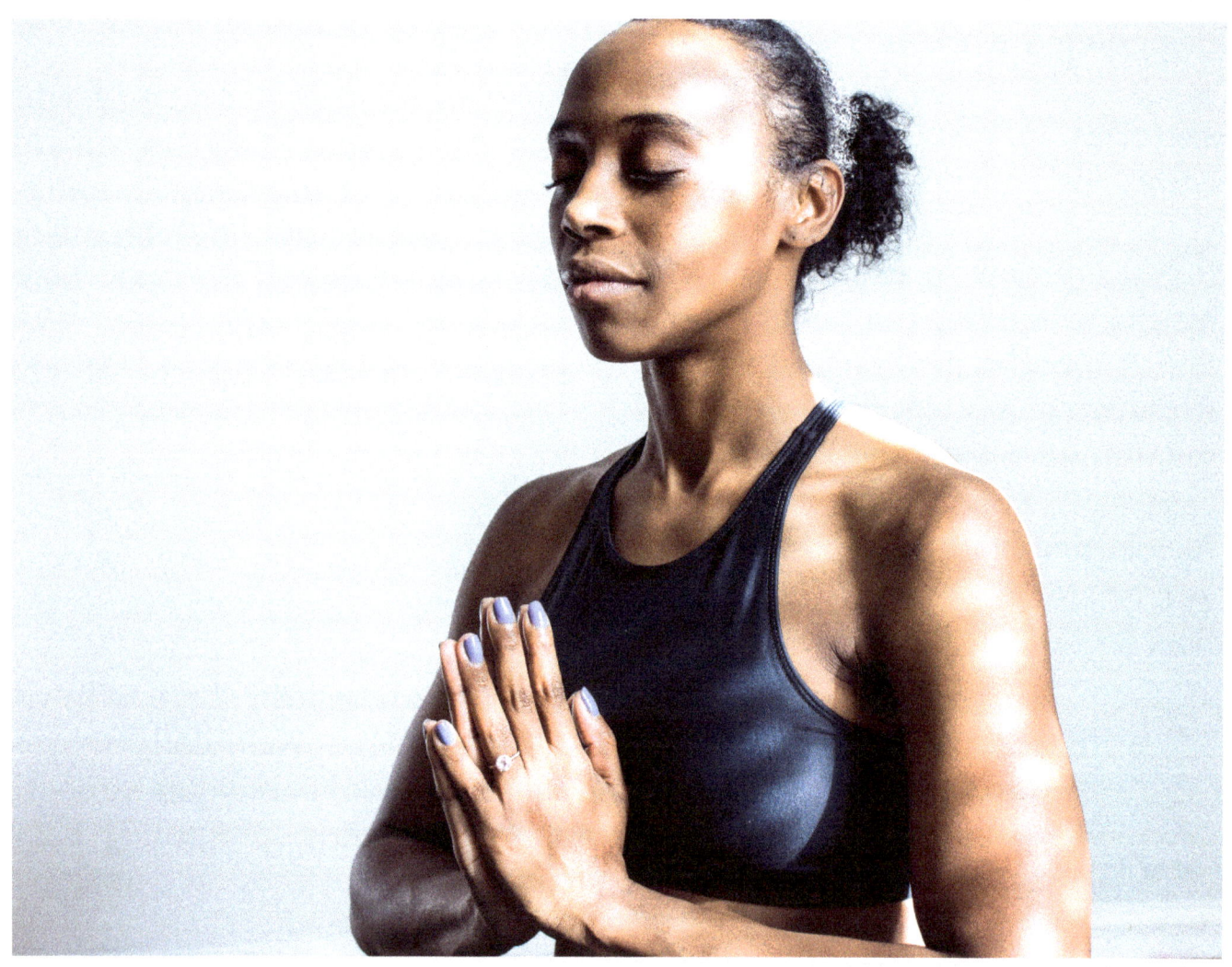

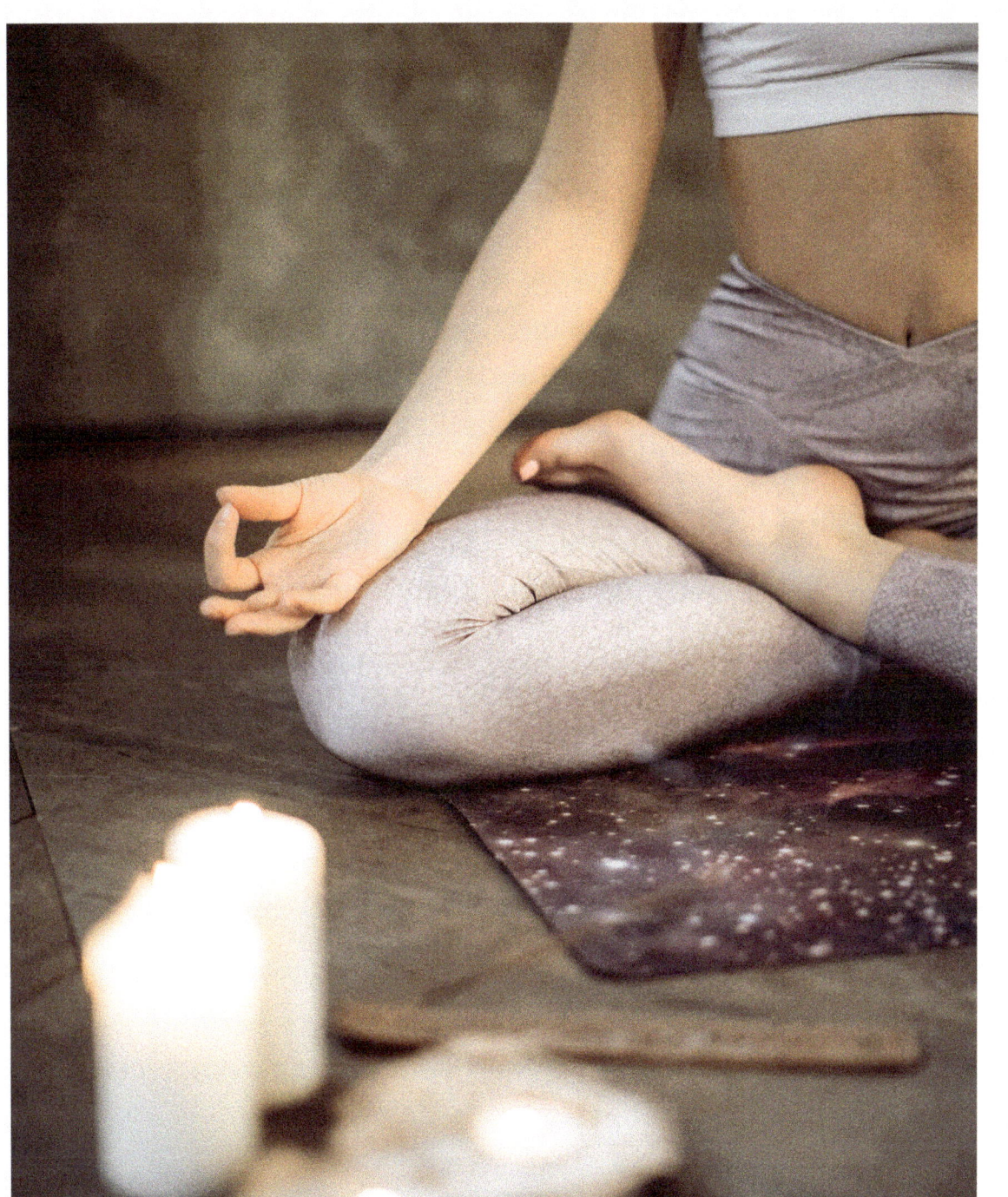

Building Foundations to Movement

Abdominal Breathing

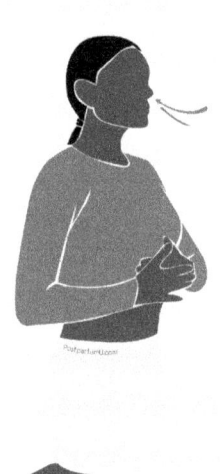

This is a technique used to engage the core. It's also an amazing tool for calming, body awareness, and resetting the vagus nerve (which controls motor function and sensory intake).

Although this is a gentle core workout that's perfect for postpartum, its effectiveness should not be underestimated.

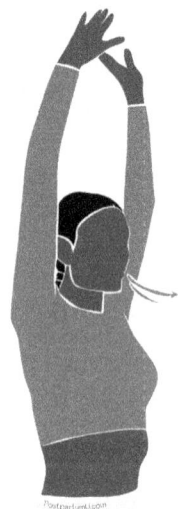

To do this exercise, breathe in deep, slow breaths. Visualize your lungs filling with air all the way to your belly button. Breathe in through your nose and exhale slowly through your mouth, being sure to push all the air out of your lungs. Breathe in again slowly, all the way to your belly button, and repeat several times in a row throughout the day.

Important Note: If you have diastasis recti or suspect that your abdominal muscles are separated, be sure that you hold your stomach muscles together while you practice this deep breathing. This way, your breaths don't cause further separation and damage.

Everything we do affects our hormones and their balance, which, in turn, affects everything we do.

Posture Awareness

When you are breastfeeding or carrying around a baby all day, your shoulders and neck fall forward. On top of having a weak core from pregnancy, your posture can take a backseat and even bring you physical pain.

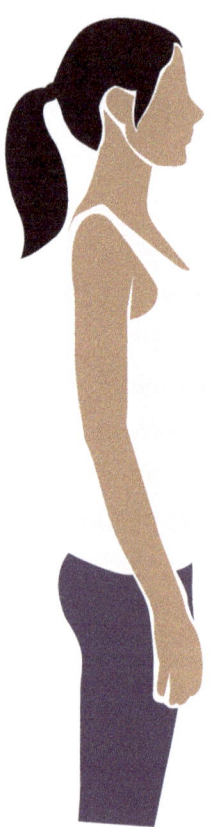

When you are sitting or standing, while holding your baby or not, practice good posture with your back straight, shoulders back, stomach in, and head level. When you do this, your muscles, especially in your core, will really feel it! Practice this every time you notice your posture decline. Consciously change your posture often. You will build up the muscles that support good posture and it'll become easier for you.

Again, if you have diastasis recti, make sure to support your core with your hands or a belly wrap (NOT a bind) that is geared toward bringing your body together in closing. The bengkung belly wrap is my personal favorite as it fits to your unique body form.

Back to the Roots

A Story from Around the World

In many parts of **Africa**, motherhood is greatly tied to that of Mother Earth. She births in contact with the earth to receive its strength. The placenta and umbilical cord are buried in the ground to give fertility back to the mother and restore her womb to good health. Many foods are considered taboo in postpartum, including fruits, sweets, and even ice. In the Congo, a mother goes back to live with her family for 3 months, where she focuses on rest, nourishment, and recovery.

Gentle Stretches

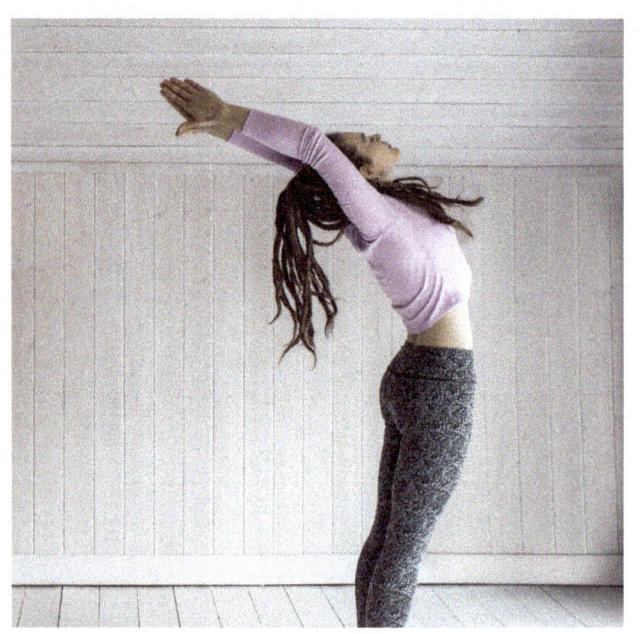

As you feel more comfortable to take on exercise, spend some time in the morning and/or evening doing gentle stretches. Be conscious of how you feel when you do this, paying special attention to not overdo it. Some of the most beneficial stretches involve laying or sitting on the floor. Not only are they gentle, they feel amazing too.

Closing Yoga

Closing yoga is a term to describe the sealing, or coming together, and "the end." These moves are typical at the end of a regular yoga session. But in postpartum, they play an important part in closing, or ending, the open bones and pelvis you've had since pregnancy. These exercises are gentle reminders for the body to return back to its normal "closed" positions, such as the pelvic bones coming back together.

Some closing yoga positions on the next page include child's pose, happy baby pose, supine spinal twists, legs-up-the-wall pose, and modified bridge pose.

Closing Yoga Positions

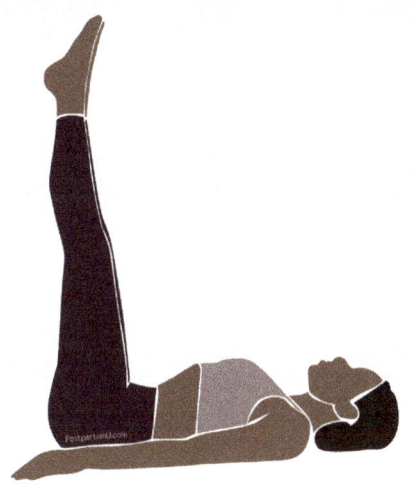

Legs-Up-The-Wall Pose

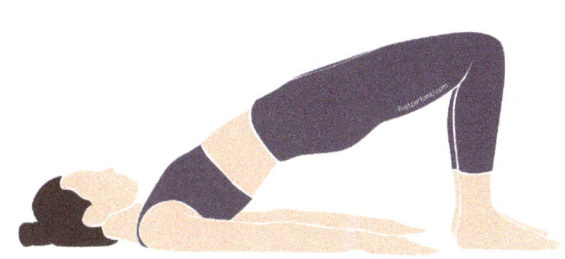

Modified Bridge Pose

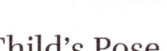

Child's Pose

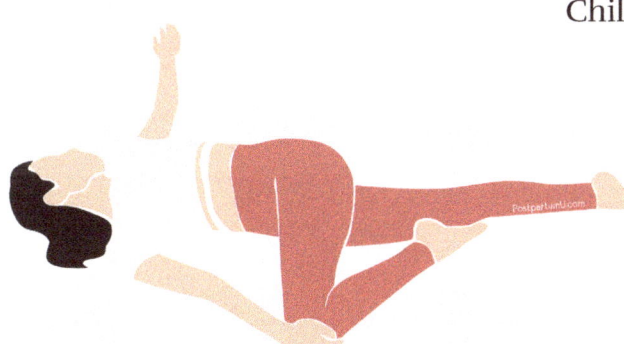

Supine Twist Pose

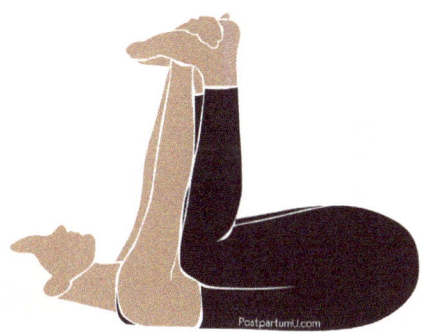

Happy Baby Pose

A Word on Cardio and Weightlifting

For many, cardio exercise, like running, is something that feels necessary. If cardio and/or weightlifting was a part of your life through your pregnancy, don't hesitate to jump back into the game (gently, of course). And if you are new to the world of cardio workouts, weightlifting, or even taking up sports, consider seeing a Pelvic Floor Physical Therapist before getting this active.

Be sure to go easy on yourself as you begin this journey into stronger workouts and check in often with your body. Reassess constantly and make sure you are feeling well. Then enjoy the benefits of working out and feeling strong.

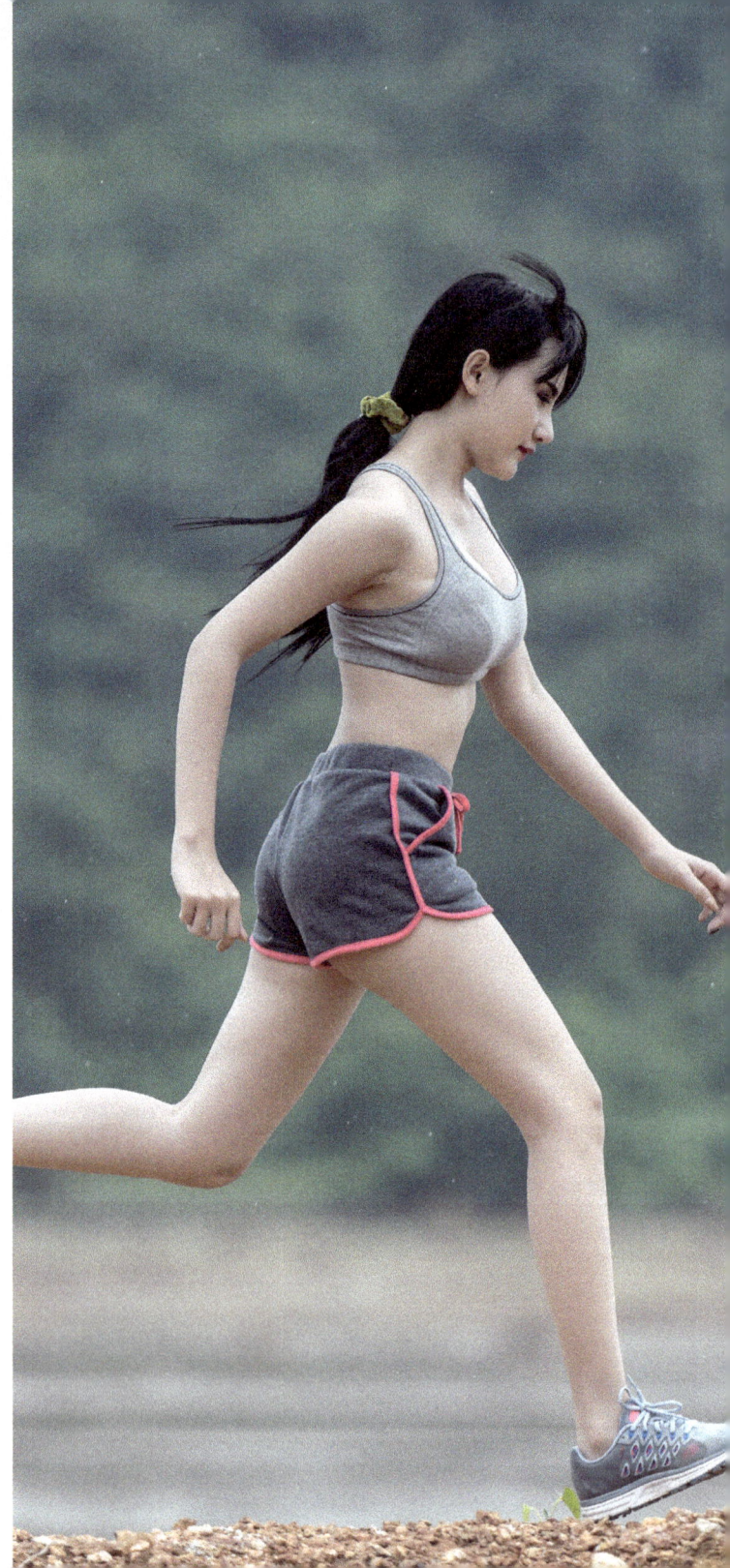

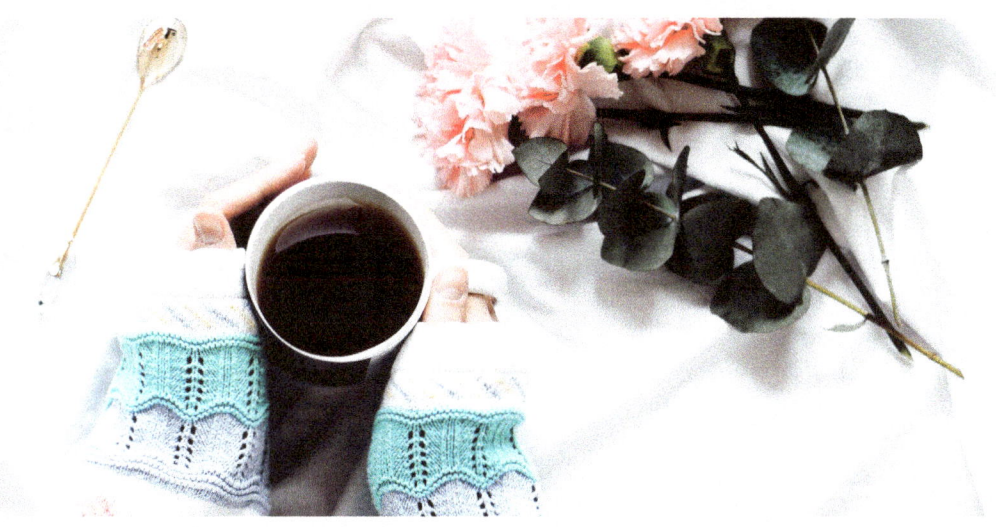

The Answer Resides Inside You

All of the strategies within this book are tools and actionable techniques that you can begin doing today to support your health and healing.

When women are fully supported on a mental, physical, emotional, and spiritual level, they radiate that to their children. As the center and creator of your life and your children, your healing carries forward to them. A healed mother heals her home, and many healed homes heal communities and the world at large.

Although this guide gives my clients a significant number of tools to support getting them off antidepressants, helping them sleep 8-9 hours rather than their standard 3-4, saving marriages, healing birth trauma, supporting healthy fertility after years of miscarriages…it is still missing a few components that I cannot provide.

The first is community. No matter how much I give you here, it may not feel easy or doable without the support of others. Motherhood is a learned experience. So is healing. In order to heal the generational wounds that have been handed to us (and to not pass them down the line), it's critical that we come together, share, and support one another through times of change.

Never has that been more clear than now.

The other part that this guide lacks - and could never fill - is the ability to do it for you. Without your action, this plan and everything within it means nothing. You must take steps to make positive change in your life and in the lives of those around you.

Remember, this is not just about you. This is about your children, your partner, and your community..and they (as well as you!) deserve health, wellness, and a life that is free of generational trauma, baggage, and habits that don't serve anyone.

This all begins with you.

With Love,

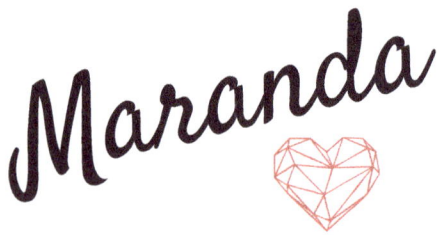

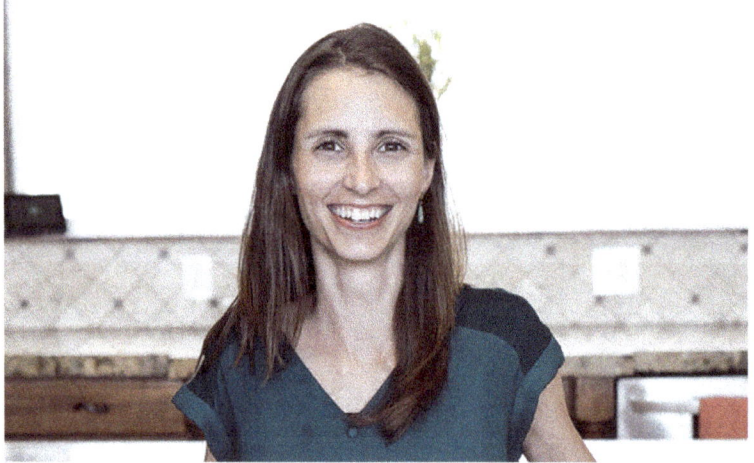

Glossary of Terms:

Art Therapy: A therapeutic technique that uses art-based exploration to enhance mental and emotional health. There is really no limit to the art forms that can be used. Although a trained Art Therapist can serve as a major benefit, anyone can engage in art as a means of healing. For more information on Art Therapy, go to www.PostpartumU.com/Workbook.

Breastfeeding Professional: There are several types of breastfeeding professionals. Whether a Certified Lactation Consultant, Lactation Counselor, or Lactation Educator, getting evidence-based support from a trained professional can help you successfully meet your breastfeeding goals.

Diastasis Recti: The separation of a pair of muscles (generally known as your abdomen). This split is common after pregnancy and can cause weak core and pelvic floor muscles, back pain, digestive concerns, and bulging that resembles bloating.

Dis-ease: The word "disease" refers to abnormalities within the body that are typically inflammatory, painful, debilitating, and even deadly. In this book, a hyphen is used to bring awareness back to the root cause of the disease itself, rather than focusing on the pathological symptoms that have people feeling as if they have little to no control over their body. Many diseases are symptoms of much larger imbalances and dysregulation that are rooted in the Steps to Postpartum Wellness found in this book. Hyphenating the word itself is to convey awareness of this fact and to refocus on bringing "ease" back into your life.

Dysregulation: In postpartum, dysregulation refers to an abnormality that brings the physical, mental, and/or emotional self into a state of confusion, chaos, or disorder. It's a disturbance to the biological systems and keeps the human body out of harmony. Long periods of dysregulation generally cause dis-ease over time.

Doula: A support person who provides ongoing physical and emotional assistance during pregnancy, labor, and/or postpartum. Generally, doulas are trained non-medical professionals with knowledge and tools to bring a mother and family comfort during the significant event that is motherhood. There are doulas that are also trained to work with mothers and families through miscarriage, death, and non-reproductive health scenarios.

Dysfunction: In postpartum, dysfunction refers to the lack of function or malfunction within the body, either with a bodily system or an organ. This is usually the beginning breakdown of the body before entering a state of dysregulation.

EMDR: Eye Movement Desensitization and Reprocessing (EMDR) Therapy is a non-evasive type of psychotherapy technique used to support individuals in healing from trauma. EMDR is a growing evidence-based therapy that is clinically effective, especially in the perinatal (pregnancy through postpartum) period.

Emotional Symptoms: A vast array of emotions that are often unwelcome and recurring. They can include sadness, anger, hopelessness, guilt, shame, anxiety, confusion, exhaustion, loneliness, lack of interest, disappointment, fear, and more. In postpartum, many of these emotions may also be intertwined with more positive feelings. These symptoms can be signs of needing further support.

Evidence-Based Science: Refers to a standard of practice that includes objective up-to-date research and data, ideally through randomized controlled trials. Preferably, this science should be applied with social, cultural, and individualized care needs and desires.

Health: A state of physical, mental, emotional, and spiritual well-being. The definition of health is also very personal and should be reflected upon by the individual. What does health mean to you?

Holistic: Considering the whole of a person, rather than the small parts that make up an individual. Derived from the word "holism," which stresses the significance of nature, holistic usually implies a more natural approach to whole body care, healing, and living.

Imbalance: In this book, imbalance refers to atypical or irregular biological processes or functions within the body. This is not to be confused with the ebb and flow of hormones, emotions, or cyclical living. Rather, imbalance is strained, and often leaves a person feeling unwell.

Intuitive/Intuition: The ability to tune into your body and know or perceive something without the constraints of societal views, personal trauma, and/or what would be deemed "facts" or "proof." Intuition is innate and can grow over time with conscious practice.

Organ Prolapse: When weak pelvic floor muscles and tissues exist, internal organs such as the uterus, bladder, vagina, or rectum descend lower into the pelvis. Symptoms can cause pressure, pain, back aches, urinary or fecal incontinence, painful intercourse, and more. If you are experiencing these symptoms or suspect that you have organ prolapse, please see a Pelvic Floor Physical Therapist.

Pelvic Floor Physical Therapist: A specialized area of physical therapy with specific training and support for those with problems related to the pelvic floor. For more information on Pelvic Floor Physical Therapists, go to www.PostpartumU.com/Workbook.

Physical Symptoms: Refers to a vast array of physical manifestations that are often unwelcome and recurring. They can include headaches, hair loss, stomach pain, gas and bloating, acne, aching joints, and more. These symptoms are a clear sign of needing further support.

Postpartum: The first several years after having a baby that encompass a physiological, psychological, and even spiritual transformation.

Root Cause Care: The act of addressing the whole body's symptoms and needs, then supporting personalized health and healing at its very core. Rather than focus on treating the symptoms, Root Cause Care looks at the whole individual and applies solutions that reach the underlying issues.

Self-Care: Anything that a person does to better their physical, mental, emotional, and spiritual well-being. It is an act that is best applied within a healthy lifestyle and supports an ongoing healthy relationship with oneself.

Sleep Training: Practices and tools that train a baby to sleep through the night. Often viewed negatively due to many methods and tools commonly used that can be harmful to a baby. Healthy biologically normal sleep training for babies and parents is possible without harsh methods that leave you feeling guilty. To find what is safe and works best for your family go to www.PostpartumU.com/Workbook.

Somatic Therapy: An evidence-based therapeutic technique designed to bring awareness to the mind and body connection. Its focus on body sensations and their connection to emotions and mental thought processes help many people with physical ailments and trauma.

Traditional Medicine: A type of medicine derived from generational knowledge and practice. Traditional Medicine consists of more organic therapies and tools derived from nature itself, well before the era of modern made-made medicine.

Trauma: An emotional response from witnessing or experiencing a difficult or stressful situation that then causes ongoing distress physically, mentally, emotionally, and/or spiritually. Not all people who experience/witness a disturbing event will have trauma. It's important to note that trauma is in the eyes of the beholder, meaning that even if something wasn't deemed traumatic for one person it doesn't mean it wasn't for another.

TRE® Therapy: Tension and Trauma Releasing Exercise Therapy® is a non-invasive technique that helps remove stored trauma within the body using shaking, a method that induces a normal biological response to high stress. You can do this along with a trained practitioner for maximum benefit, and you can learn to do this exercise yourself in the comfort of your home by going to www.PostpartumU.com/Workbook for more information.

Whole-Body Healing: See "holistic."

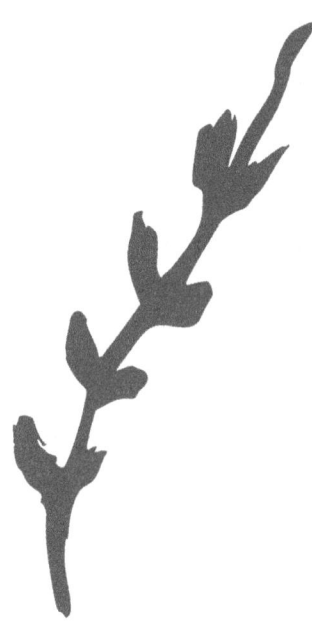

Acknowledgements

No amount of words could express my deepest gratitude for all that have supported me through the creating and birthing of this book. Just as in birth and postpartum, it has taken a village of support to create, and I simply cannot forget this labor of love and all those who were present for it.

For my husband and children, who've been my light and my spunk and my reason for nearly all that is good in my life...

For my ancestors. Those who have paved the path and shared with me insights and wisdom beyond my own capabilities...

For my incredible team: Tiffany Grierson and Megan Schoenleber, without your hard work and support in the creation this book, it wouldn't even be here. Seriously, it would be nothing but a Word document and a dream...

For every mother, child, and family. For being my greatest influence to keep going, for your kind words, and for your encouragement to keep going even when I thought giving up was the best option...

For all those I cannot begin to mention here... For the encouragement, enlightenment, the wisdom, resources, conversations, time, attention, and love you have shared with me, it hasn't gone unnoticed.

Thank you.

Additional Resources

This book is simply the beginning! For more visit:
www.PostpartumU.com/Workbook

Postpartum Recovery Assessment:
www.PostpartumU.com/Quiz

Free Postpartum Nutrition Handouts for Professionals:
www.PostpartumU.com/Handouts

Postpartum Nutrition Plan:
www.PostpartumU.com/Nutrition

Postpartum Nutrition Certification for Professionals:
www.PostpartumU.com/Certification

Postpartum University Podcast:
www.PostpartumU.com/Podcast

References

Aghajafari F, Letourneau N, Mahinpey N, Cosic N, Giesbrecht G. Vitamin D Deficiency and Antenatal and Postpartum Depression: A Systematic Review. Nutrients. 2018; 10(4):478. https://doi.org/10.3390/nu10040478

Barba-Müller, E., Craddock, S., Carmona, S. et al. Brain plasticity in pregnancy and the postpartum period: links to maternal caregiving and mental health. Arch Womens Ment Health 22, 289–299 (2019). https://doi.org/10.1007/s00737-018-0889-z

Beck CT, Watson S, Gable RK. Traumatic Childbirth and Its Aftermath: Is There Anything Positive? J Perinat Educ. 2018 Jun;27(3):175-184. doi: 10.1891/1058-1243.27.3.175. PMID: 30364308; PMCID: PMC6193358.

Chauhan G, Tadi P. Physiology, Postpartum Changes. [Updated 2020 Dec 8]. In: StatPearls [Internet]. Treasure Island (FL): StatPearls Publishing; 2021 Jan-. Available from: https://www.ncbi.nlm.nih.gov/books/NBK555904/

Craig WJ. Nutrition concerns and health effects of vegetarian diets. Nutr Clin Pract. 2010 Dec;25(6):613-20. doi: 10.1177/0884533610385707. PMID: 21139125.

De Punder K, Pruimboom L. The Dietary Intake of Wheat and other Cereal Grains and Their Role in Inflammation. Nutrients. 2013; 5(3):771-787. https://doi.org/10.3390/nu5030771

Dennis, C. L., Fung, K., Grigoriadis, S., Robinson, G. E., Romans, S., & Ross, L. (2007). Traditional postpartum practices and rituals: a qualitative systematic review. Women's Health, 3(4), 487-502.

Eisenberger, N., Moieni, M., Inagaki, T. et al. In Sickness and in Health: The Co-Regulation of Inflammation and Social Behavior. Neuropsychopharmacol 42, 242–253 (2017). https://doi.org/10.1038/npp.2016.141

Elaine S. Barry, James J. McKenna. Reasons mothers bedshare: A review of its effects on infant behavior and development; Infant Behavior and Development, Volume 66, 2022, 101684, ISSN 0163-6383. https://doi.org/10.1016/j.infbeh.2021.101684.

References

Etebary S, Nikseresht S, Sadeghipour HR, Zarrindast MR. Postpartum depression and role of serum trace elements. Iran J Psychiatry. 2010 Spring;5(2):40-6. PMID: 22952489; PMCID: PMC3430492.

Frances A. Champagne, James P. Curley. Epigenetic mechanisms mediating the long-term effects of maternal care on development. Neuroscience & Biobehavioral Reviews, Volume 33, Issue 4, 2009, Pages 593-600, ISSN 0149-7634, https://doi.org/10.1016/j.neubiorev.2007.10.009.

Hansen MM, Jones R, Tocchini K. Shinrin-Yoku. (Forest Bathing) and Nature Therapy: A State-of-the-Art Review. International Journal of Environmental Research and Public Health. 2017; 14(8):851. https://doi.org/10.3390/ijerph14080851

Haus, E., Touitou, Y. (1992). Principles of Clinical Chronobiology. In: Touitou, Y., Haus, E. (eds) Biologic Rhythms in Clinical and Laboratory Medicine. Springer, Berlin, Heidelberg. https://doi.org/10.1007/978-3-642-78734-8_2

Hunt J. R. (2003). Bioavailability of iron, zinc, and other trace minerals from vegetarian diets. The American journal of clinical nutrition, 78(3 Suppl), 633S–639S. https://doi.org/10.1093/ajcn/78.3.633S

J. P. Lallès, Long term effects of pre- and early postnatal nutrition and environment on the gut, Journal of Animal Science, Volume 90, Issue suppl_4, December 2012, Pages 421–429, https://doi.org/10.2527/jas.53904

Jodi R. Godfrey. Toward Optimal Health: Robert J. McConnell, M.D., Discusses the Clinical Opportunities for Improved Thyroid Disease Management in Women. Journal of Women's Health. May 2007. Volume: 16 Issue 4. 458-462. http://doi.org/10.1089/jwh.2007.C074

Karakula-Juchnowicz, H., Rog, J., Juchnowicz, D. et al. The study evaluating the effect of probiotic supplementation on the mental status, inflammation, and intestinal barrier in major depressive disorder patients using gluten-free or gluten-containing diet (SANGUT study): a 12-week, randomized, double-blind, and placebo-controlled clinical study protocol. Nutr J 18, 50 (2019). https://doi.org/10.1186/s12937-019-0475-x

References

Kendall-Tackett, K., Cong, Z., & Hale, T.W. (2011). The Effect of Feeding Method on Sleep Duration, Maternal Well-being, and Postpartum Depression. Clinical Lactation, 2, 22 - 26.

Khashan AS, Kenny LC, Laursen TM, Mahmood U, Mortensen PB, Henriksen TB, et al. (2011) Pregnancy and the Risk of Autoimmune Disease. PLoS ONE 6(5): e19658. https://doi.org/10.1371/journal.pone.0019658

Kim, Pilyoung, Leckman, James F., Mayes. et al. The plasticity of human maternal brain: Longitudinal changes in brain anatomy during the early postpartum period. Behavioral Neuroscience, Vol 124(5), Oct 2010, 695-700.

Laura E. Sockol. A systematic review of the efficacy of cognitive behavioral therapy for treating and preventing perinatal depression. Journal of Affective Disorders, Volume 177, 2015, Pages 7-21, ISSN 0165-0327, https://doi.org/10.1016/j.jad.2015.01.052.

Leslie M. Swanson, Heather Flynn, Jennifer D. Adams-Mundy, Roseanne Armitage & J. Todd Arnedt. (2013) An Open Pilot of Cognitive-Behavioral Therapy for Insomnia in Women with Postpartum Depression, Behavioral Sleep Medicine, 11:4, 297-307, DOI: 10.1080/15402002.2012.683902.

Lester BM, Conradt E, LaGasse LL, Tronick EZ, Padbury JF, Marsit CJ. Epigenetic Programming by Maternal Behavior in the Human Infant. Pediatrics. 2018 Oct;142(4):e20171890. doi: 10.1542/peds.2017-1890. PMID: 30257918; PMCID: PMC6192679.

Marc G. Berman, Ethan Kross, Katherine M. Krpan, Mary K. Askren, Aleah Burson, Patricia J. Deldin, Stephen Kaplan, Lindsey Sherdell, Ian H. Gotlib, John Jonides. Interacting with nature improves cognition and affect for individuals with depression, Journal of Affective Disorders, Volume 140, Issue 3, 2012, Pages 300-305, ISSN 0165-0327, https://doi.org/10.1016/j.jad.2012.03.012.

McGee, M., Bainbridge, S., & Fontaine-Bisson, B. (2018). A crucial role for maternal dietary methyl donor intake in epigenetic programming and fetal growth outcomes. Nutrition reviews, 76(6), 469–478. https://doi.org/10.1093/nutrit/nuy006

References

Mørkved, S., Bø, K. The effect of postpartum pelvic floor muscle exercise in the prevention and treatment of urinary incontinence. Int Urogynecol J 8, 217–222 (1997). https://doi.org/10.1007/BF02765817

Mulraney, M., Giallo, R., Efron, D., Brown, S., Nicholson, J. M., & Sciberras, E. (2019). Maternal postnatal mental health and offspring symptoms of ADHD at 8-9 years: pathways via parenting behavior. European child & adolescent psychiatry, 28(7), 923–932. https://doi.org/10.1007/s00787-018-1254-5

Mulraney, M., Giallo, R., Efron, D., Brown, S., Nicholson, J. M., & Sciberras, E. (2019). Maternal postnatal mental health and offspring symptoms of ADHD at 8-9 years: pathways via parenting behavior. European child & adolescent psychiatry, 28(7), 923–932. https://doi.org/10.1007/s00787-018-1254-5

Nelson, C, & Carver, L. (1998). The effects of stress and trauma on brain and memory: A view from developmental cognitive neuroscience. Development and Psychopathology, 10(4), 793-809. doi:10.1017/S0954579498001874

Osteria T. S. (1982). Maternal nutrition, infant health, and subsequent fertility. Philippine journal of nutrition, 35(3), 106–111.

Peden, A.R., Hall, L.A., Rayens, M.K. and Beebe, L.L. (2000), Reducing Negative Thinking and Depressive Symptoms in College Women. Journal of Nursing Scholarship, 32: 145-151. https://doi.org/10.1111/j.1547-5069.2000.00145.x

Peden, A.R., Rayens, M.K., Hall, L.A. and Grant, E. (2005), Testing an Intervention to Reduce Negative Thinking, Depressive Symptoms, and Chronic Stressors in Low-Income Single Mothers. Journal of Nursing Scholarship, 37: 268-274. https://doi.org/10.1111/j.1547-5069.2005.00046.x

Prescription Medicine During Pregnancy. March of Dimes. July, 2022. https://www.marchofdimes.org/pregnancy/prescription-medicine-during-pregnancy.aspx

References

Redpath, N., Rackers, H. S., & Kimmel, M. C. (2019). The Relationship Between Perinatal Mental Health and Stress: a Review of the Microbiome. Current psychiatry reports, 21(3), 18. https://doi.org/10.1007/s11920-019-0998-z

Rockers, P., Sharda, A., & Shet, A. (2019). Maternal Malnutrition, Breastfeeding, and Child Inflammation in India (P11-025-19). Current Developments in Nutrition, 3(Suppl 1), nzz048.P11-025-19. https://doi.org/10.1093/cdn/nzz048.P11-025-19

Roux, G., Anderson, C., & Roan, C. (2002). Postpartum depression, marital dysfunction, and infant outcome: a longitudinal study. The Journal of perinatal education, 11(4), 25–36. https://doi.org/10.1624/105812402X88939

Sarah E. Hall, Matthew Beverly, Carsten Russ, Chad Nusbaum, Piali Sengupta. A Cellular Memory of Developmental History Generates Phenotypic Diversity in C. elegans. Current Biology, Volume 20, Issue 2, 2010, Pages 149-155, ISSN 0960-9822, https://doi.org/10.1016/j.cub.2009.11.035.

Satyanarayana VA, Lukose A, Srinivasan K. Maternal mental health in pregnancy and child behavior. Indian J Psychiatry. 2011;53(4):351-361. doi:10.4103/0019-5545.91911

Song C, Ikei H, Miyazaki Y. Physiological Effects of Nature Therapy: A Review of the Research in Japan. International Journal of Environmental Research and Public Health. 2016; 13(8):781. https://doi.org/10.3390/ijerph13080781

Trujillo EB. Effects of nutritional status on wound healing. Journal of Vascular Nursing : Official Publication of the Society for Peripheral Vascular Nursing. 1993 Mar;11(1):12-18.

Ullrich, P.M., Lutgendorf, S.K. Journaling about stressful events: Effects of cognitive processing and emotional expression. ann. behav. med. 24, 244–250 (2002). https://doi.org/10.1207/S15324796ABM2403_10

Waldmann A, Koschizke JW, Leitzmann C, Hahn A. Dietary iron intake and iron status of German female vegans: results of the German vegan study. Ann Nutr Metab. 2004;48(2):103-8. doi: 10.1159/000077045. Epub 2004 Feb 25. PMID: 14988640.

References

Waynforth, D. (2007), The influence of parent–infant cosleeping, nursing, and childcare on cortisol and SIgA immunity in a sample of british children. Dev. Psychobiol., 49: 640-648. https://doi.org/10.1002/dev.20248

Yehuda, R. and Lehrner, A. (2018), Intergenerational transmission of trauma effects: putative role of epigenetic mechanisms. World Psychiatry, 17: 243-257. https://doi.org/10.1002/wps.20568

Yu-Ling Tsai, Chien-Chih Chiu, Jeff Yi-Fu Chen, Kung-Chi Chan, Sheng-Dun Lin. Cytotoxic effects of Echinacea purpurea flower extracts and cichoric acid on human colon cancer cells through induction of apoptosis. Journal of Ethnopharmacology, Volume 143, Issue 3, 2012, Pg 914-919, ISSN 0378-8741, https://doi.org/10.1016/j.jep.2012.08.032

More detailed and comprehensive list of references is available within Postpartum University®

www.ingramcontent.com/pod-product-compliance
Ingram Content Group UK Ltd.
Pitfield, Milton Keynes, MK11 3LW, UK
UKHW050852280725
7097UKWH00057B/1572